MINDFUL THERAPEUTIC
CARE FOR CHILDREN

of related interest

Why Can't My Child Behave?
Empathic Parenting Strategies that Work for Adoptive and Foster Families
Amber Elliott
Foreword by Kim S. Golding
ISBN 978 1 84905 339 6
eISBN 978 0 85700 671 4

Communication Skills for Working with Children and Young People
Introducing Social Pedagogy
3rd edition
Pat Petrie
ISBN 978 1 84905 137 8
eISBN 978 0 85700 331 7

A Short Introduction to Attachment and Attachment Disorder
Colby Pearce
ISBN 978 1 84310 957 0
eISBN 978 1 84642 949 1
Part of the JKP Short Introductions series

Empathic Care for Children with Disorganized Attachments
A Model for Mentalizing, Attachment and Trauma-Informed Care
Chris Taylor
Foreword by Peter Fonagy
ISBN 978 1 84905 182 8
eISBN 978 0 85700 398 0

Child Well-Being
Understanding Children's Lives
Edited by Colette McAuley and Wendy Rose
Foreword by Dame Gillian Pugh
ISBN 978 1 84310 925 9
eISBN 978 0 85700 393 5

Supporting Traumatized Children and Teenagers
A Guide to Providing Understanding and Help
Atle Dyregrov
ISBN 978 1 84905 034 0
eIBSN 978 0 85700 391 1

Games and Activities for Exploring Feelings with Children
Giving Children the Confidence to Navigate Emotions and Friendships
Vanessa Rogers
ISBN 978 1 84905 222 1
eISBN 978 0 85700 459 8

Working with Children and Teenagers Using Solution Focused Approaches
Enabling Children to Overcome Challenges and Achieve their Potential
Judith Milner and Jackie Bateman
ISBN 978 1 84905 082 1
eISBN 978 0 85700 261 7

MINDFUL
THERAPEUTIC CARE
FOR CHILDREN

*A Guide to
Reflective
Practice*

DR JOANNA NORTH

Jessica Kingsley *Publishers*
London and Philadelphia

Every effort has been made to trace copyright holders and to obtain their permission for the use of copyright material. The author and the publisher apologise for any omissions and would be grateful if notified of any acknowledgements that should be incorporated in future reprints or editions of this book.

First published in 2014
by Jessica Kingsley Publishers
73 Collier Street
London N1 9BE, UK
and
400 Market Street, Suite 400
Philadelphia, PA 19106, USA

www.jkp.com

Library of Congress Cataloging in Publication Data
North, Joanna, 1957-
  Mindful therapeutic care for children : a guide to reflective practice / Dr. Joanna North.
    pages cm
  ISBN 978-1-84905-446-1
  1. Cognitive therapy for children. 2. Meditation--Therapeutic use. 3. Child psychotherapy--Philosophy.
  I. Title.
  RJ505.C63N67 2014
  618.92'891425--dc23
                              2013024161

British Library Cataloguing in Publication Data
A CIP catalogue record for this book is available from the British Library

ISBN 978 1 84905 446 1
eISBN 978 0 85700 840 4

Printed and bound in Great Britain by Bell & Bain Ltd, Glasgow

CONTENTS

ACKNOWLEDGEMENTS

This book was originally written as a teaching manual for my team at the children's home that I opened in 2012. Therefore, I have to acknowledge some very special people who helped me out at that time and really did hang on to their mindfulness even though times were challenging for us. These are Dean Walters, Gerry Tomlinson, Steve Butchart and of course my daughter Sophie North and my husband David Wright who worked with me. These people have my love and gratitude for going through a difficult time with me but still maintaining their respectful attitude and dignity. My thanks and love, go to Jayne Smith (and her partner Helen) and her business partner Heather Broad of Crossways Care who later took over my children's home and made it their own. These women have my admiration for the complex work that they do with children and young people, and I will think of them forever as more than just business colleagues because of their kindness to me.

My supervisor last year was Dr Nick Sarra and I think he is great at encouraging reflective practice, but he is also just a lovely human being who has been kind and inspiring. Mary Roddick is a family therapist who has supported me for five years by supervising my work, and I thank her for helping me to think more broadly and more clearly. The editor of this book is Steve Jones from Jessica Kingsley. This man has insight! He spotted the potential in my original poorly written and careless working manual that was originally designed to help my team towards reflective practice. I would also like to thank my friend Dr Janine Braier who has supported me in my career development this year and who has been able to remain mindful and loving towards me even at a time of the most extraordinary challenge in her own life. I have many supportive friends who chose to understand me, and my life is the richer for it.

Most of all I am so lucky to have had at all times, unswerving loyalty, love and constancy from my husband and daughter. Their unambiguous, unfaltering love for me is so obvious and I am lucky to have them in my life. Thank you both for believing in me. David is now freer to play some extra rounds of golf and my daughter Sophie is now a psychotherapist for the future generation – determined to encourage self-expression in others and live a creative and productive life.

This book really acknowledges children and young people who feel misunderstood and who may feel that they are very alone. I hope that this book encourages someone somewhere to give you that extra moment that gives you hope and helps you to reflect on creating a beautiful life for yourself in spite of the adversity you have experienced. Don't ever give up. Your brain can start afresh every day.

PREFACE
A NOTE ON THE WRITING OF THIS BOOK

The idea for this book arose in the course of researching the best ways to care for children with complex behaviour for my doctorate in psychotherapy. I arrived at what struck me as a crucial point in my learning: that the carer state of mind is the biggest influence on changing a child's style of relationship.

It is the single factor in moving an infant with an anxious and insecure attachment forward to a secure attachment. The work of Hodges and Steele has found that maternal states of mind affected the development of previously maltreated children (Hodges, Steele *et al.* 2003) and this idea is underscored by the neuroscientific work of Schore who talks about child development as a mind on mind experience – i.e. the parental mind is the only tool for the development of the child's mind (Schore 1994).

The Wait, Watch and Wonder project focuses on developing a parent's sensitive responses to infant behaviour (Cohen *et al.* 1999). I took this hypothesis and worked with sets of parents and carers who were struggling to secure the behaviour of their previously maltreated children. We worked on the premise that our own state of mind would be the key to change (North 2010). This piece of research did not offer any amazing quick fix techniques, but I discovered that it was hard work on the part of carers, especially when children were older and had suffered from significant harm. I now offer advice to parents and carers, who often ask me for 'the next technique'. I have to say, 'no – we are out of techniques.'

My proposal is a hard proposal. It focuses on the way that we manage ourselves on a daily basis while we deal with the difficulties that children bring to us, either through their behaviour or through their communication.

How do we maintain a sensitive and responsive stance that helps children to process difficult information about their lives? This book represents the work that I have carried out since that first piece of research, exploring the best skills for managing states of mind, and drawing extensively on mindfulness skills. For example, I have been impressed by the work of Williams, Teasdale, Segal and Kabat-Zinn on mindfulness and depression (Williams *et al.* 2007): many of the carers I work with fall into despair and resignation when faced with the relentlessness of complex behaviours presented by children who have been maltreated and abused. It is only through working through these states of mind that we find our equilibrium, retain our integrity, and find the space to pause and make sense of what it is we are encountering.

Chapter 1

INTRODUCTION

This book is designed to support the development of reflective practice skills and the art of giving meaning to experience, particularly in the complex task of therapeutic childcare and caring for vulnerable children. It draws on 20 years of knowledge and experience in working with young people who are in need of a high level of support and care, particularly with behavioural difficulties, in addition to work as a psychotherapist with children who are placed in the care system. It is written for anyone trying to achieve change and support in direct work with children, whether engaged in a team within a childcare charity, a manager, counsellor, therapist, social worker, foster carer, childminder, teacher, teaching support worker or adopter, or indeed a nurse or doctor taking care of vulnerable children in hospital.

Whatever your role, the book aims to provide an introductory guide to some of the ideas that lie behind reflective and mindful practice – offering 'building blocks' in the form of information to help you increase the quality of your knowledge and thinking, and in doing so increase the quality of your practice.

A key aim of the book is to increase the quality of reparative childcare: to help you to develop a useful skill set and focus of mind. By using the information and tools in this book you should be able to increase your capacity to think through tough issues, as well as develop a confident capacity to notice and capitalise on the moment-to-moment experiences and emotions essential to the task of understanding children.

Reflective practice and mindfulness has much to benefit children. It is important for us to gain greater understanding of children who struggle with accepting the care and authority of adults and who have complex behaviours. However, if adults cannot understand how they themselves work, they are unlikely to understand or be a model of behaviour for children who are lost and bewildered.

Unless we as caring adults model our expectations through our own behaviours then we are giving nothing, sending messages which may be contradictory and are not gaining the respect of young people. Children are born to notice instantly the behaviours of adults, and will register straight away whether you say what you mean and do what you say. Children copy and mirror – they are programmed to do this, and their brains are powerful mirrors of the mental and emotional environments in which they live.

So carers have to examine the values, attitudes and the beliefs that they impart in their day at work with children and young people. In caring for children carers are not just doing a job, they have taken up a vocation in which there is a need to constantly develop skills and expertise in oneself. The first foothold towards this goal is that carers can reflect on their experiences and learn from them. The second is to understand that, if you are more adept at understanding yourself, then you will transfer this learning to young people who in turn will grow to understand themselves.

It is also essential that practitioners start to understand the communications that children are constantly making through their behaviour to us as adults. If we become proficient at noticing behaviour in children we will be able to help them make sense of, and give meaning to their own behaviours, and in turn help them to increase the management of their behaviour as well as their communication skills.

If we can do this, children may no longer have to engage in acting out painful experiences in an attempt to communicate their pain.

Any guidance has to recognise just how difficult this can be on the ground; events can change and emotions shift. When working with difficult children who are ensnared in a difficult frame of mind, carers can quickly get lost in the quicksand of chaos of mind, and lose their clarity of thought and positive intentions. More often than not a dysfunctional environment can ensue, and a group of well-meaning carers can become stuck at the lowest end of the spectrum of possibility. All human beings are capable of desperation, fear and extreme rage. We have to show that we can manage these behaviours in ourselves.

So, I am promoting the simple idea that awareness of how you are will help your self-management skills, and help to regulate your system so that you achieve a more attuned state of awareness through reflective practice. More than this, it has the potential to transform the environment in which you work.

These are simple steps to creating optimum work with children. They are steps that require absolutely no money whatsoever, but they do require some time set aside for both reflective and mindfulness practice, either in a group or on an individual or one-to-one basis, and they do require some commitment to the idea that reflective practice is useful. This book is designed to describe exactly why reflective practice will be useful to you.

THE BOOK'S PHILOSOPHY AND INFLUENCES

In writing this book, I have drawn on a mixture of approaches, professional fields, philosophies, theories and ideologies including psychology and psychotherapeutic and psychoanalytic theory and neuroscience in order to understand better how our minds work.

It is my belief that we learn more effectively by drawing on useful ideas, whichever particular field of study they originate, and this relates to the stance of the book as a whole – to encourage open thinking.

It is increasingly accepted that one particular model or theory, used exclusively and in isolation from all other fields of information, is likely to lead to a closed and inward-looking system. A typical example of this would be the way that psychoanalytic theory has become more accessible since absorbing the information from research on the function of the attachment relationship.

Psychologist John Bowlby, who developed attachment theory, was initially rejected and isolated from the field of psychoanalysis because of his scientific approach, and spent many years tolerating this status.

His book *Childcare and the Growth of Love* was controversial when published for public consumption in 1953, based on a report he authored for the World Health Organization called 'Maternal Care and Mental Health' in 1951. It asserted that the baby or child needs to experience a warm, intimate and continuous relationship with his or her mother (or permanent mother substitute) in which both find satisfaction and enjoyment, even though at that point there was little research to prove it. At the same time, he began to think of psychoanalysis as hopelessly unscientific.

However, an eventual melding of the two fields that once were actively in opposition to each other, and a breaking down of the barriers around knowledge, has provided a broader sphere of information from which to understand children.

The approaches outlined are also influenced by the European model of social pedagogy which invites a high level of engagement between carer and young person in order to yield the best results for that young person in terms of their social learning. Social pedagogy places an emphasis on the quality of the relationship created between carer and young person, and the carer has a vocation to teach and coach the child about how to cope with the social world and how to manage relationships.

John Bowlby articulated clearly the connection between primary relationships or parents and attentive care in infancy, and mental health and well-being in adulthood. His theories have been tested over 50 years, and more recent research in neuroscience and neurobiology tend to prove him right (notably the work of neuroscientists Alan Schore and Dan Siegel, which will be covered later).

Another key theory associated with reflective practice is Action Learning as developed by Reginald Revans (Revans 2011) which can be used to increase organisational productivity. If you are engaged in reflective practice in your work then you have created a learning environment or a learning organisation (Senge *et al.* 1999). This means that you are likely to learn as quickly as possible from your mistakes and not repeat them, so that you are always changing and adapting in the best possible way.

Another disciplinary division in recent times has been that between the behavioural approaches of cognitive behavioural psychology and psychotherapy, which is often seen to be at odds with relationship psychotherapy and the attachment model of personality development which focuses on relationship. However, in focusing on the mind, this book argues that as both fields of information are part of the same continuum of the development of the brain, and the brain is both relational as well as cognitive in its functioning, there is value to be found in both approaches.

This book is intended to provide a combination of theory and practice (praxis) in conjunction with a reflective stance, to provide a model for a sensitive, measured and creative response to children's needs – we can learn much from experience and theory. More than anything children need the accurate and sensitive attention of compassionate adults who understand them and who are able to withstand their difficulties.

Working with children can be done on an individual basis, as part of a group, or as a combination of individual and group work. The material that follows recognises the richness of diversity and difference as well as the power of working together. Humans have developed with a paradox in that they can be both randomly individualistic as well as deeply social animals.

I believe that we function at our best when we are 'both and' rather than 'either or' creatures.

As well as providing information to encourage a reflective outlook, I include in Chapter 6 a model – the 'Reflective Practice Pentagon' which is intended to be a tool box for the art of caring – to help understand or conceptualise the lives and difficulties that young people experience.

The overall aim is to develop reflective practitioners who are able not just to act, but also to think and plan and to 'keep their heads when all about them are losing theirs' (Kipling 1895, p.83) in the firm conviction that it is our thinking or at least the way we manage our thinking that is the crucial element of this work.

As a starting point, in Chapter 2 I have identified some of the underlying values of reflective practice.

SUMMARY

- Reflective practice requires a set of skills, and the ability to interpret our experiences and give meaning to the behaviours of others in order to find solutions to difficult scenarios.

- Through reflective practice we can increase the quality of our thinking and the quality of our experience, and transfer this into our work with children and young people.

- Being open to many sources of information can influence our practice in positive ways, and encourage open thinking. We can be informed by established theories like attachment theory (Bowlby 1953) at the same time as theory from the social sciences such as social learning theory, and social pedagogy. We can also be informed by philosophy, art, music and poetry.

- The ultimate goal is to be well-managed, self-regulated, thoughtful and sensitive carers.

Chapter 2

BEING REFLECTIVE AND REFLEXIVE

This chapter describes some of the underlying values and frameworks of reflective practice. These are not strategies just for psychotherapists, they are skills for anyone wanting to improve their own communication skills and help others: the tools we can use and develop when caring for children therapeutically in an effort to put their lives on an even playing field; giving them the same opportunities to communicate in a way that secure and well-loved children can.

First, the terms: it helps to understand what it means to be reflective or reflexive.

BEING REFLECTIVE

To be reflective is a natural process of the working of our minds. It is the capacity to think about experience and relationships and organise units of meaning so that it makes sense to us. Peter Fonagy has called this process Reflective Functioning (Fonagy and Target 1997).

It may help to see this as 'tidying the rooms of the brain' so that we are ready for the next set of experiences – putting away toys after a day's play or organising files in the filing cabinet. It is what we all do regardless of IQ or life experiences; it is a function of the flow of energy of the brain. The brain always likes to work its way towards its most regulated and organised state, so that it is in an optimum position in order to be prepared for the next set of experiences. Sleep is another great opportunity for the brain to organise itself and we notably do this through dreaming and deep sleep. We awake refreshed and the problems with which we have gone to bed may not seem so acute because the brain has been organising experience.

Reflective functioning can be seen as a vital process that takes place unconsciously. The brain is all the time organising itself. This tendency works regardless of class or faith and is an equalising factor in human functioning. We all have this capacity. You might be a little bit more fortunate if your parents helped you to be reflective about life – but not necessarily. People who have had very bad and highly incoherent and disorganised experiences in life can be reflective and the good news is that it can help you to get on with your life. You can learn to be reflective even if you do not have this as an innate part of your behaviour.

Peter Fonagy (Fonagy and Target 1997) who developed a measure of reflective functioning, noticed that the capacity to reflect can assist in putting right things that may have gone wrong or been difficult because we can mentally tidy the cupboard and start again. We can make links with our past in order to make sense of current behaviour. This is the first reason why I think it is important for us to be reflective more consciously and to learn about this process. Our brain is busy organising anyway; we could be more conscious of this, and that would mean we are more mindful.

BEING REFLEXIVE

Reflexivity on the other hand is about our capacity to think about the outside world and the impact that the different layers of our social world have on our thinking and experience. If we are reflexive in our thinking it means we are noticing the many institutions of our society, including those which are apparently invisible. This extends to noticing our environment: the ecosystem and the tectonic and geographical evolution of the globe – these all impact on us too and we certainly get to know about them when we witness an earthquake followed by a tsunami as we saw in Japan 2011. That is reflexivity. The better we are at it, the more it can help us.

Reflexivity is the ability to consider the impact of different layers of our lives upon experience. It is based on our knowledge of the world and the way that it works through us. Being more conscious of this may help us to gather more information more quickly, to note how the world impacts on us. If we are reflexive we will anticipate things before they happen.

For example, a child's behaviour may be difficult. Your ability to think about the way that affects you emotionally and mentally is an act of reflection. If you go further and consider the impact of the economic system, the social care system, the parental home conditions on the child – that is an act of reflexivity. Reflexivity is a conscious effort to take thinking further and be aware of 'other' or outside factors. An exercise to enhance this would be to stop for a moment and think about all of the external factors that impact on your life. For example, you could ask yourself – what impact does religion have on my life? Even if you are an atheist, you will have some answers to this question.

In terms of brain development the capacity to be reflexive is part of more mature development. Pre-schoolers are delightfully unaware of the impact of the outside world, junior school children are delightfully inaccurate about the impact of outside factors, whereas teenagers tend to think they know the impact of everything in their lives yet their knowledge base may fall short of the mark on occasion. Reflexivity can be acquired knowledge and so it is possible to increase your capacity to be reflexive.

So far so good. However, we may have experienced resistance to being reflective or reflexive at times. This particularly occurs when we are busy and thinking logically all the time, or focused on the 'doing' mode of life as is often the case in children's care homes or indeed ordinary homes. I attended a seminar by Dr Ruth Leitch (Leitch 2010) when she offered us the opportunity to reflect on our unconscious selves through the use of art. We were to bring a shoe box and craft items to decorate the box – the final product would be called a self-box and would be a representation of ourselves both conscious and unconscious.

As I am unbelievably bad at art, I won't describe the finished product in detail except to say that I finished with boxes within boxes with fancy ribbons, bows and decorated paper. I could not have been less interested at the outset of the project. I was so busy working six days a week and writing a doctorate in psychotherapy – 'What could be the point for me?' I thought, 'I know who I am.' I had forgotten to bring a box and craft items, and so Ruth Leitch lent me a shoe box. I just happened to have some old photos in my bag and I borrowed sticky tape and glue, and delved into the pile of craft items. I was attracted to ribbons and brightly coloured paper. The outcome of that session was that I realised that I had actually forgotten myself through having so much work to do and the self-box was a symbol of my forgotten self.

Having run similar sessions since that day, I know a common first reaction is, 'This is so boring and why doesn't she get a life and what has this got to do with our work – I just got kicked by an angry child last night and it hurts.' And then people will get on with their collage or picture and will make the breakthrough that says – 'Aaaah, OK. I've got it – there is another way to think about this and there is a whole other layer of me. Can we do more of this reflective thinking – it's such a relief.' Some other part of our brain is at work – actually working for us and not against us – the organising, reflective aspect of the brain which is just dying to get a look in!

I have been moved by the number of staff teams who have been willing to make the breakthrough in their resistance to thinking and reflecting at another level, even when they have felt initially resistant. Some of the thinking and emotion that can be expressed through art work and pictures can be truly inspirational – sometimes in its simplicity and sometimes in its complexity. However, it is possible to increase the functioning of the reflective aspect of the brain simply by looking for pictures that inspire you. A simple picture from a newspaper or magazine is enough to provoke reflective thought. A collection or scrapbook of such pictures would be a wonderful opportunity. A mood book or picture board for a team would be a great focus for the team and a reminder to stop and think. Equally, listening to music can offer a perfect opportunity for reflection and integration.

Without opportunities for reflection, our work is simply a set of activities without any considered meaning. However, the more important issue is that in stopping for reflective practice we have enabled ourselves to think more holistically, more accurately and we will have more information about the scenarios we are facing. We will be able to think clearly both for ourselves and for the children we care for, and just maybe we will influence them to be able to think more reflectively, giving meaning to their experience and making it safer to reflect, because we have made the ground safe by our own example.

Children who have been raised in neglectful and pathogenic homes have not had parents who have helped them communicate their inner lives and organise experience into meaningful memory. Often deeply chaotic experiences crash into each other time and time again in these children's lives and as a consequence they present us with minds that are chaotic, out of control, apparently lacking in meaning and sometimes just dangerous. Trauma, fear and learned dysfunctional behaviours mean that these children will act out time and time again. It takes enormous reserves and a lot of courage on the part of a carer to hold fast and help these children to realise that the mind can regulate their experience, and that adults can be helpful and are not all harmful. In order to be more successful in achieving positive outcomes for children and young people, carers have to learn better ways to help children feel safer and think more clearly. Reflective practice is what can take us there.

REFLECTION AND BEING EMOTIONALLY LITERATE

Ignoring your own emotions can be seriously disabling, as in reality your emotional response to life is your friend – talking to you and telling you about your authentic minute-by-minute experiences and giving you feedback. It is how you manage your responses to your emotions that matters, not how you successfully eject, eliminate and ignore your emotions. So, it's important to listen carefully to your inner lives at this level. This is 'emotion regulation' and it is the key to happy living in that an emotional state tends to help us to organise and integrate thinking. It gives richness and colour to the world, helping the mind to link its various functions and flow in a more fluid fashion. Without emotion, it's likely that our own responses will be mechanistic and rigid.

Our basic emotions include sadness, fear, anger, shame, surprise, disgust and joy. These categories are universal, found across all ethnic groupings and cultures and are unique to human beings and their communication.

We read emotions in people all the time and we are usually watching their faces for their immediate responses in order to achieve this reading. Emotion is an expression of a state of mind and is also a physiological or bodily response to our experience, so emotion links both body and mind. Think for example if you are laughing – how much you feel that in your face, your throat and your stomach and even your legs and feet. You cannot laugh and be stressed at the same time. If you are crying or in grief, you might notice how much sadness you can feel in your heart or chest, and you might stop eating because your nervous system is primed to serve the emotion first.

Emotional states reveal what is really in our mind, giving depth to our lives and linking us with our instinctive and mammalian selves. The primary emotional state of fear served to keep us safe, priming our systems to be ready for fight or flight millions of years ago. We have not lost that primitive base to our emotions despite the fact that our minds are more evolved. When we are expressing emotion, we are at our most human and perhaps at our most vulnerable, and also at our most accurate in sharing our communications. More than anything, all emotion is healing for the mind. Think how much better you feel after a good cry about something with which you are struggling or upset. The feeling of release occurs as the chemical balance changes when we stop trying to control our response after some upset, we then feel accepting and peaceful.

The brain can re-organise itself after the tears and shuddering of grief; we can find equanimity and the mind returns to its harmonious state. We accept our experience as it is (Siegel 2012a). Without emotional expression our mind can become inflexible and we can prevent ourselves from being informed by experience and knowing ourselves well. It is so very important that we value our own emotions and the emotional communications of children in particular. That does not mean you have to be indiscreet about your emotions – it is quite right that emotions are a private matter most of the time, unless we choose to share them. I must correct a common fallacy that people who express emotions are showing some instability. It is far more likely that people who know their emotions well and can manage them well are likely to be attempting to stabilise themselves on a regular basis and are therefore well-balanced people. People who are emotionally accurate themselves are often more empathic to others. They are also perceived to be authentic in their communications, and authenticity is a trait that is noted to be high on the list of things that are most liked about people who are popular.

Through counselling and being heard, people can become more aware of their inner lives and the value of emotional states that have previously been a nuisance to them. People come to counselling saying, 'Can you help me get rid of this state?' So often they will leave having learned to live with and welcome their states of mind – that is of course as long as those states are ultimately manageable and not overwhelming for too long. Those who have not been so aware of emotions need have no fear of this idea. By being aware of the general principle that emotions are a mode of valid communication, you can start to notice the states of others and give those states some value. We will thus be more effective and more helpful to others – supporting children to manage their overwhelming emotions – because we have mastered the art of understanding and regulating our own emotions.

There are some notable exceptions to emotional literacy, in that some children or adults quite organically find attention to the emotional self quite difficult. For example, children with autism spectrum disorders (ASD) are often described as having a 'triad of impairments' of social communication, social imagination and social relationships. While each individual child is different, children with ASD tend to have a very linear concept of life – it is not helpful to try and 'force' them to enjoy their emotions, or consider them to be odd because they do not. However, that doesn't mean that one cannot help such children considerably in being able to make sense of the emotions of others.

On the whole it is good practice to support children on the autism spectrum to consider the idea that other people do have emotions and are functioning on this level. Autistic spectrum children and adults can become isolated and unhappy if their world view is misunderstood, and can feel rejected.

ASD commonly involves difficulty in processing feelings. Most people can work out what someone is thinking and feeling by looking at their face and using sensory systems to sense their communication. Children with ASD find this very difficult. They will give very literal meaning to most communications – they hear the words and try to construct a picture according to the words that they hear, but may fail to find another layer of meaning.

They also find it difficult to imagine what it would be like to be like someone else (theory of mind). As a result they can be undiplomatic, appear to be insensitive and uncaring, and they can unwittingly sound stunningly rude or arrogant. They often have a special area of interest in which they are engrossed. These subjects vary, and they may include complex categories involving detailed classification or alternative science fiction worlds. Children with ASD can be extremely focused on their subject, and it can be hard to move them away from this in conversation.

So, clearly we are not all the same in our communication styles, but remember this does not mean that communication is not happening. Be aware that not everyone will revel in creative reflective practice or expressing emotions – be reflective about how such adjustments might be made, and seek out information where you need it. In the case of working with children with ASD, I'd recommend familiarising yourself with the work of Professor Simon Baron-Cohen at the Autism Research Centre of the University of Cambridge (Baron Cohen 2001).

REFLECTION AND COMMUNICATION

Reflective practice is a way to increase our communication both with ourselves and with others. However, you do not have to be a good communicator to engage in the art of reflective practice. We are not all great masters of communication and sometimes it takes some time for us to realise that communication is happening anyway regardless of our efforts to suppress it.

For example, if we stand smoking a cigarette at tea-break time, hoping for some respite, a moment of recovery, what are we actually doing? We are really communicating with ourselves and the cigarette facilitates a sense of calm and provides some soothing – a moment of respite. That cigarette is an expression of something, a need in yourself. In this moment of quiet therefore, we are responding to the deeply seated impulse of self-preservation – one of the constant communications from the seat of the mind to the self. Sitting quietly then can be as valuable in communication as sharing a torrent of ideas.

Equally, drawing a picture or cutting out a picture from a magazine can be as informative as chatter – often far deeper and more informative. We may be drawn to a picture but not know why – perhaps it's the colour or the tone or the shape or perhaps it prompts a memory or deeply held belief about life – but either way if it is worth our attention then the picture is communicating something to us. This is why I often encourage silent reflective practice sessions where participants are invited to plough through magazines and newspapers so that they can pull out ideas that impact on them. Frequently in these kinds of sessions I find that participants start off chattering and enjoying a read of the papers, they then gradually become very quiet and very engrossed as they find something emerging from their search – a story or a picture that attracts their attention. Participants then build their own collage based on this material. Even the sceptics can find something to put down on paper.

In these kinds of artistic reflection we can find ourselves, just as we can find ourselves if we walk by the sea or cook something wonderful or even in smoking a cigarette quietly (although I recognise the complexity in finding respite in a cigarette with regard to health). As you work through this book you will realise that we all have a form of self-expression, and that children most certainly are trying all the time to communicate – even if it is in some perverse or awkward way through behaviour or in some way that makes us want to run away from them. It is the richness, texture and shape of our ideas that matter and the courage to bring ideas to the surface and give meaning to experience which is important.

REFLECTING ON EQUALITY AND POWER

I once had an argument with a friend. It was upsetting and it took me a long time to think about that argument and what it meant. Ultimately I realised that my great discomfort with the whole communication with him was the fact that he did not see me as his equal. He did not say this, but it emerged in the communication between us as he amply demonstrated that my opinions were disregarded as well as discarded. I knew instinctively that what I had said was of no value to him – I felt that *I* was of no value to him. This made me angry. We recovered from the argument – as people do recover from disagreements. But the question I was left with was – why does equality matter so much?

Equality matters so much because power matters so much. And whilst we may live in a democracy (if we are fortunate enough) that pays much attention to the narrative of equality – that does not mean that we live in a country that is equal. We do not. As I said to my beloved friend, 'A goldfish is always the last to know about water.' By this I was pointing out that he was a white male in a senior position of power both through his profession and his senior years who was unaware of any sense of what it was like to feel unequal to him. Consequently he made me feel unequal simply through his presence – without even trying.

People who are fortunate enough to have a handful of power in this life may well want to stop and consider the impact of this power over people. Power may come through your designation before your name (i.e. Lord, Lady, Doctor), it may come because of financial power; you may have power because you have celebrity status or because you have a particular skill, or indeed because you are the biggest, strongest person in the room and are therefore perceived to be physically more powerful. You may also have power because you were born with it – i.e. into a titled position that assumes power and authority – such as that of a Lord (a position which is currently under consideration at a political level in this country due to the absurdity of the rule of primogeniture by which men inherit the title and not women).

I refer to this deep source of inequality in the United Kingdom in particular because it demonstrates very amply the depths of our historical inequality – it also shows that we have come a long way to try and equalise opportunities. Whatever the source of power in your life or indeed whatever the source of disempowerment in your life (and it is for sure that we will have both senses) we really do need to communicate on the basis that we are equal in our ability to communicate. This of course particularly becomes important when we work with people who are vulnerable and desperately disempowered. Power becomes something tangible – it becomes a set of ideas and it becomes an energy that actually flows through our lives. People with learning difficulties should be helped to be on an even playing field with those who have sufficient cognitive ability. They can then communicate their needs in just the same way as those who find this easy. If we are not helping those who are disempowered and if we are not conscious of the chasm or shadow that inequality can cast in communication, then it is likely that we will make unwitting errors in our care and in the assumptions that we make about children and young people.

Children and young people have one deep disadvantage in life – they have no power over adults. It is true that they grow towards autonomy and they develop their sense of equality but as infants, toddlers, pre-schoolers, in middle childhood and early, mid and even late teens, ultimately they are not in control of what happens next. At best, they have a sense that the adults who care for them will listen to them and receive their communications and be mindful of their position. We forget just how disempowered and vulnerable children can feel simply by virtue of their chronological or developmental disadvantage. Unfortunately children who have no sense of management or control due to poor communication skills will often act out the insecurity this causes them through violence and aggression as a way to seek control. Of course they are rejected because of this, and few people take into consideration the root cause of aggression in children and young people. Children are usually acting on an instinct and that instinct is 'If we are not equal then we are not safe'. If children do not feel safe they are likely to react in primitive ways to keep themselves safe.

Equality then is the first act of civilisation, giving rights to all of us in equal measure and most certainly the right to feel safe. We have seen this principle develop over the history of civilisation – slavery, once commonplace, is now a crime although clearly not eradicated altogether. Acts of racial discrimination or genocide of races are legislated against, although again this primitive tendency to eradicate those who are 'not like us' is not yet purged from the world that we live in. If man and womankind are not given the tools to be equal then we will resort to animal behaviour which dictates that the stronger (and most powerful) will survive and the weakest will not have the same freedom as the strongest and will live in fear of them. It only takes a moment of reflection to think this through to a logical conclusion – this sort of power dynamic does not work, or at least only for the few. Women would be afraid of men because they are encoded to be stronger and our whole society would be built on a framework of power and fear. If we are going to communicate effectively and give more vulnerable people an equal playing field so that they feel more secure, we have to get our equality consciousness together. The act of functioning reflectively does not encourage the acquisition of power through force – it requires that we look further to understand and give meaning to the causes of behaviour, particularly in the children we care for and in the groups of people we work with. I have developed this idea in the Appendix where I have reproduced The Rights of the Child as espoused by the European Convention on Human Rights. It is helpful reading and is certainly a focus for our ideas and concepts of equality during reflective practice.

SELF-ACCEPTANCE

I talk about the self and its significance to reflective practice in more detail in Chapter 5 of this book. Ultimately acceptance of self and others will radically change the way your world is working, because it will change the way your brain is working.

As fallible humans we have an innate tendency to reject and drive away that which we do not like. We often do not like things that are very different from us. This works as a protective mechanism, keeping us safe. Something that is alien to us may well be able to destroy us – a dinosaur would have most certainly worked along this principle. However, we have evolved since this time. However, it could still be considered foolish not to run away from the things that we fear or the people we dislike. In reflective practice our instincts are trained and honed to go in the other direction. We are trained to face up to what is going wrong and to face down our frightening demons which usually present themselves in the form of the judgements that we make about situations.

If our judgement about a child we are caring for is that they are 'evil' then we are most certainly facing a demon that is our own. If we stop, pause and think for a while, wading through the information that is available to us about a child's behaviour, taking guidance from the minds of others, we are much more likely to formulate conclusions that make it possible to work with such a child rather than abandon them. If your formulation about a child is that 'she is doing it on purpose' then you are bound to feel vengeful and even vindictive. If you can gradually see that children, even if they do something on purpose, in fact are just crying out for attention and trying to communicate, then you are likely to behave in more productive and constructive ways. This is not to say that we cannot make judgements to keep ourselves safe. If a child is coming at you with a knife – this is not the time to sit and reflect – it is the time to get out of the way. Later is the time to give meaning to a child with a knife. So the underlying principle, if you are working reflectively, is that ultimately you are going to move towards an acceptance of a child and their behaviour, rather than a rejection and that this acceptance will bring some radical changes in that behaviour.

From this acceptance of the child you are likely going to have to change your stance towards many other people including yourself. You may have to start to accept some of your own demons, tendencies and anxieties. If you are able to offer this same acceptance and understanding to yourself then you will fill the pool of self with more energy, more self-esteem and a lot more happiness. In rejecting ourselves, which we seem more easily geared to do, we leave a void inside that makes us fragile and leaves us separated from others. We try to avoid this shame, embarrassment and sense of unworthiness. Instead of understanding that we are all vulnerable to shame through our mistakes, we make ourselves feel isolated and alone. The fact of the matter is that we are all vulnerable to mistakes both at work and in our personal lives and that shame is a human emotion and an inevitable aspect of what will go on inside us. Through a process of reflection we can give meaning to our mistakes, accept the inevitable discomfort of some shame and then move on to make the necessary changes.

SUMMARY

- **Reflective and reflexive practice.** Some people use the terms reflective and reflexive synonymously to mean the way in which we 'think about our thinking' or the way in which we give meaning to and interpret our experience, but this book defines reflective as engaging in the act of thinking about our thinking reflectively, and reflexive practice as a behaviour that involves reflection on several levels.

- **Emotional literacy.** Reflective practice involves being conscious of how our brain works in conjunction with our emotions. Emotion is a great part of our intelligence. The more we pay attention to it through mindfulness and emotional literacy, the more accurate we will be in our understanding and interpretation of children's responses to us.

- **Equality.** Equality is important and vital to reflective practice because it can help us to interpret both what is right and wrong about the world that we live in and allows us to reflect on power dynamics.

- **Acceptance**. If you work reflectively you will move towards acceptance of a child and their behaviour and that this will bring about some radical changes in that behaviour.

Chapter 3

BEING MINDFUL

Mindfulness is at the heart of reflective practice. Being mindful involves being in touch with your own mind and the constant flow of information and energy that flows in waves through your brain, as well as the brain of every other person around you.

There is nothing at all mysterious about being more aware of how your mind works – in fact it could be seen as an act essential to your survival. It is sometimes seen as an act of religion or spirituality – a connection often made with mindfulness practice due to its past association with Buddhism and the ancient art of meditation and contemplation. However, mindfulness does not have to be associated with religion in any way for it to work.

Why is it important to know more about the way our minds work? Precisely because we are able to influence the activity of our minds, and for our minds in turn to influence how we behave.

Dan Siegel, author of *The Mindful Therapist* (2010a) asks the question, 'what is a mind?' He notes that most people – even brain experts – don't have a clear definition of their own mind, but in his book Siegel provides a useful answer to the question:

> Mind relates to our inner subjective experience and the process of being conscious or aware. In addition,

> mind can also be defined as a process that regulates the flow of energy and information within our bodies and within our relationships, an emergent and self organizing process that gives rise to our mental activities such as emotion, thinking and memory. (Siegel 2010a, p.1)

It is particularly illuminating to think about the mind in these dynamic terms in connection with work with young people, whose minds are still in the process of development. At this stage it is possible to make changes or repair behaviour.

It's also interesting that Siegel talks about 'flow', as reflective practice is all about concentrating on the flow of information and energy both in our minds, our lives and in our work.

We share information and energy in all of our relationships – whether in the workplace or at home, and it could even be argued that at its root, life is a process of sharing information and energy. We are working with our own mind and the minds of others in a continuous flow, and in the case of children, their minds are even more fluid and less rigid as they develop and form a mind of their own.

Siegel proposes that the mind is to be found both in the brain – the machinery of the mind – but also in relationships with others (Siegel 2010a). The expression 'we are of the same mind' can be seen as an expression of this. Relationships are critical to who we are: they mirror our own minds, determine our development when young, and are the way we share information and energy with one another. What is life if we don't share information and energy?

Relationships play a significant role in therapeutic work and therefore attention to the quality of the communication and interaction needs to be given priority. In addition to this we need to focus on the climate of the emotional environment in which the young person exists, including our own state of mind, the state of mind of the young person and the team around the child.

Similarly, if we are not sharing information and energy through relationships, we lack flow and become blocked and cut off from one another. Our thinking becomes more rigid and less open to influences for change; the same principle applies to groups and organisations. A blocked organisation will result in disorganisation, chaos, excessive rigidity, institutionalisation and unhappiness. When the blockage bursts the outcome can be a chaotic explosion, catastrophe or critical incident where information and energy is quickly scattered in all directions and we wonder how to begin to organise the flow.

Siegel uses 'harmony' to describe the potential state of our minds: at its most settled and most functional the mind is harmonious – like a song which is in tune (Siegel 2010a, pp.31–32). Try engaging in an act of mindfulness right now in order to give attention to the mind – perhaps put the book down and sit quietly for a moment and ask yourself the question, what is the tune of my mind? Or what range of tunes reflect your state of mind?

My own tunes tend to range from Stravinsky's very untuneful, unharmonious and fretful 'The Rite of Spring' at one end of the spectrum to the Paul McCartney song 'Let it Be' at the other depending on the time of day and the pressure that I have allowed myself to be under.

By carrying out the simple act of thinking about the tune and rhythm of your mind, you will have come to know yourself better. You are more aware of the workings of your own mind and therefore yourself.

The things that take place in our lives, brains and minds could be viewed as a striving to return to harmony or a state of comfort and regulation.

There are many words that describe this tendency to restore a state of balance so that we can live our lives most effectively. People are not at their most effective when in a state of disharmony and chaos; they cannot see their goals clearly and disharmony leads to anxiety, mental pain and stress. To think about it in evolutionary terms, someone lacking in harmony fundamentally feels they are not surviving well and that organisation is needed. This again is mindfulness.

Another neuroscientist, Alan Schore, studied how the mind develops in his book *Affect Regulation and the Origin of the Self* (Schore 1994). He clearly states that the brain develops best in infancy within the parental environment with interpersonal interaction, and that the best state of mind for parents to offer for the development of the child is that of 'joy' combined with consistent kindly, harmonious interaction and attention.

This gives us some very clear rules about the mind. The mind needs to be in relationship with others in order to develop: it needs a sense of organisation, it thrives in a state of harmony and is most productive or primed when engaged in positive emotional states.

Siegel (2010a) in his book *The Mindful Therapist* describes what may be termed as 'soft skills', which he better describes as 'essential skills, skills of introspection or skills of intersubjectivity' (Siegel 2010a, pp.4–5) as they are essential to human survival and relate to our inner world as well as our outer world.

He talks about the flow of the mind – as if it is a river of flowing water – and the flow having five aspects to it:

1. being flexible

2. being adaptive

3. having a tendency to aim towards a coherent state

4. having the capacity to facilitate an energetic flow (i.e. not sluggish and murky)

5. being stable, having essential machinery that prefers to be in a stable state.

So the mind is flexible, adaptive, coherent, energetic and stable, summarised by the acronym 'FACES' flow (Siegel 2010a).

He also asserts the two extremes of the mind – one rigidity, the other chaos and suggests that we are trying to set our thermostat somewhere in between for a healthy mental state. Too much rigidity might give us depression, too much chaos would give us uncontrolled tendencies of mania.

We will probably all recognise that some scenarios call for our control and vigilance – crossing the road with a group of pre-schoolers? Other times call for 'manic' behaviour in order to meet an important deadline – a looming inspection of our service or meeting a deadline for publication. In a healthy state the mind can manage both of these eventualities, but can very well be pushed to its limits. On the whole though we would all need to return to a balanced state of flow, equilibrium or regulation.

Think here for a minute on how many activities you employ in any one day for your mind to return to a balanced state of flow: it might be smoking, taking a coffee break or having a drink at the end of the day – all of which are socially sanctioned behaviours for relaxing and return to a more joyful and hopeful state that enables better flow. For others it may be sitting quietly or chatting and engaging in something that does not involve stress such as reading a magazine. Sometimes a trip home on the bus or the train could be a chance to relax and let go and let the mind re-assimilate after the pressures of a long day where demands are constant. These are acts of integration and regulation – simply allowing time for the mind to regain its balance.

If we know about this need of the brain to have time to return to a harmonious state we can actually ensure that we meet this vital biological and psychological need in a more conscious way.

It is most successfully met by taking time out, relaxing and consciously allowing the brain to return to its old friend – harmony. Such a simple change as giving time for reflection could be life changing and brain changing and enhance well-being. How many environments have you worked in where you have had permission to take time out and say, 'I am doing nothing so that I can help my brain.'

I will wager that it is not many. Some time last year I was training a team in reflective practice and we undertook a very simple mindfulness exercise for half an hour which included time out to rest the brain. There was a little resistance to the idea at first, but gradually the team realised that as they took time out they could feel their minds responding and a sense of well-being emerging. They liked this. By the end of the exercise they were able to note that they felt more inspired, more energised and productive and hopeful. They had managed to shift some of their worries on to a written list and they had found some harmony. They also started to think very creatively about how they could work with some very difficult children who had enormous life problems. That process involved some very simple acts which are listed below.

A MINDFUL EXERCISE

- Find a warm, comfortable place to sit where you can relax and where you are not interrupted by the phone.

- Make a list of the tendencies of your thoughts. Here is a rough guide to the kind of tendencies that could be flowing through your mind: worry, anxiety, upset, planning, scheduling, anticipation of future events, lists of things to do, frustration about past events, despondency about how to cope, annoyance at being asked to take time out of a busy schedule. All states are valid. You are the only person who gets to see this list. The aim of this is to take note of your scattered attention and gradually focus your mind.

- Make notes of any immediate matters that need your attention once you have taken this time out, i.e. you can do them in about half an hour and not before. This is a time for reflection and not doing. Put the list to one side for doing later.

- Now find an object on which you can focus your mind (that is give your attention to) – you may look at scenery out of the window or focus on a simple object like your watch. However, it is an object you are looking at to focus your attention – not the list you have just made.

- As you focus your attention on this object, allow your body to relax. You may 'slump' if it helps but just ensure that your body becomes comfortable.

- As you do this notice your pattern of breathing. You are still focusing on your object. You are engaged in focusing on an object to keep your attention in one place and just noticing the rise and fall of your breath as you do this. Notice how thoughts emerge (i.e. more aspects of the daily work of your brain such as, shopping, predicting, anticipating) but just allow these to flow away unless it is a particularly urgent thought that you may have to write down.

- Continue with this restful experience of noticing your breathing, relaxing, noticing thoughts as they continue to run through your mind for some minutes until your time for mindfulness is complete. The flow of thinking continues and you let your thoughts flow away – unless they are urgent for your to do list.

- Your initial exercise in mindfulness is complete.

You could build on this exercise by taking time out in your life and developing your ability to focus your mind – giving it time to re-energise and reharmonise. The organisation who engaged in this practice session with me now have this practice as part of their daily working lives. It is considered to be part of the culture to 'take time out'.

MIND AND BODY

The mind is situated in the body and not just within the brain. We take in information from the environment through our senses – our hearing and feeling, our touch, taste and smell and this information and energy is fed into the brain through the body from the senses via the brainstem and organised into the various 'stations' of the mind.

Therefore our bodies are very much part of our mind. Take for example the way you might experience sadness. Do you feel a pain in your brain? No you crease up from the stomach and your shoulders fold forward, and if you are really sobbing you shudder and hunch and tears stream from your eyes. If you are really laughing you laugh from the centre of your body and 'collapse' into laughter. If you are shocked or surprised the hairs on your arms and head prickle and your mouth might open with your breathing automatically becoming quicker and deeper so that you can take in more air in order to prepare for danger.

So if we are trying to think about what may be our mind – it is helpful to consider the body and the significance of the body's environment.

The brain is a master at giving meaning to experience. This is the process of 'integration', sorting all the different information we receive into a coherent whole. To name a few, the brain links information about our feelings and moods, information about keeping our system regulated, cognitive functioning, survival impulses, body functioning, memories, our immediate environment and so on. The output from all of this organised information needs to be coherent to us. There is an almost unbelievable amount of activity and we still do not have a full map of the brain's functioning.

Increased awareness of the flow of energy and information in the brain is helpful to us. If we are more conscious of our own particular brain patterning and tendencies we are more able to manage the processes of our daily lives and experience and in fact can become more effective. So the simple act of taking half an hour out to do nothing except focus our attention on how we are and what we need helps us to integrate experience, give meaning to our lives and generally regulate this flow of energy.

To give an example of the brain's capacity for integration and coherence, consider a parent caring for a toddler.

The toddler's mind/brain is mostly developed in the region of their primitive 'relational' brain. They have not yet grasped fully the concept of time frames which will come later as they develop their cognitive functioning – highly activated in our modern world so dependent on timing. There will be indicators that their cognitive brain is sparking into action as they begin to represent their experience through language. However, the toddler's brain and stage of development has an emphasis on relationship and involvement with a main carer. The main carer has to keep their attention on this aspect of the toddler's functioning in order to support them and help them to feel secure. At the same time the carer's cognitive brain has to keep a focus on the clock and the demands of the social world. It is easy to see how a toddler may be distressed or feel lost with a parent who is constantly stimulated by demands from the outside and social world. In fact they only really know the demands of their relational brain and their need for the focused attention of that parent. Any parent of a child of this age has to be able to straddle and integrate these two worlds with great sensitivity for their child, understanding their developmental stage whilst at the same time keeping their mind alert to the social world and their own needs. It can be a tricky dance and it's easy to see how a parent can obscure the relational needs of their child if they are under pressure themselves and not able to give time and thought to how to work those differing agendas from two minds.

Apply the same principle to work with complex cases and children who are needy, confused and disorganised, whose behaviour is incoherent and lacking in integration. In order to help them it really matters how caring adults effectively integrate the demands on their time with giving the child the reparative attention that they need. Within the act of reflective practice we allow some light into our own thinking so that we can understand these conflicts and mange these different worlds.

As a result of monitoring and modifying your mind through reflective practice you can increase the capacity of the brain to function. Here is another simple example. There are two sides to the brain – the left hemisphere and right hemisphere. The left side of the brain concentrates on all things that are more linear. Siegel (2010a) suggests we could remember this as 'L' for left and linear and lists. 'L' is also for language because we know that the left side of the brain is starting to 'come on line' when a child develops language at the age of two. At this age, they start to formulate the idea that everything in the world has a name, and also that questions can be asked through the term 'Why?' They realise that it is particularly useful to ask an adult those questions, as they may be able to give answers. Having this knowledge can help us not to be annoyed with them for asking continual questions – they so want to know about life and they are simply doing what their brain tells them to do now.

The right side of the brain has the task of attending to our relationships and I remember this as 'R' for right and 'R' for relationships. The relational brain develops before the left side and we are born with this right side firing away so that the child can become an expert at relating. The right side particularly attends to communication through body language and facial gestures which can be seen in the act of newborns searching for faces as a way of interacting with their very new world. Babies just love to see a face. Some of us may have an ability to utilise every aspect of left and right hemispheres of the brain – some may employ more linear thinking and some may lean more to artistic and creative ways of expression. Either way it is useful to know that we function in these left and right hemispheres and that we can be aware of different aspects of ourselves and how we can balance the different demands placed on us.

The brain has a very smart way of being friends with both the left and right hemispheres – through integration it can link knowledge from the linear left side of the brain with the creative aspects of the right side of the brain in a harmonious way so that we have optimum functioning. This energetic tendency to integrate is helpful to consider in relation to reflective practice. A well-crafted piece of poetry (using language and creativity) could be seen as the harmonious outcome to a left and right integration of the brain. You could consider how pleasing it is to hear a familiar poem and how this might help you to feel that life has meaning and that something is complete in the world. This may be very soothing to you. Similarly drawing a picture may be a way to solve a relationship problem that is causing you worry. It could be a way of bringing into consciousness some aspect of the relational side of your brain that you need to express in your life now – and may help you to think more clearly about a complicated relationship.

MINDFULNESS AND THE GROUP

Reflective practice attempts not only to link the different aspects of the brain and mind, but also to link with other people around us. This could be seen as operating in a similar way to how the brain processes experiences, through integration.

Integration as a group is crucial to create harmony. This harmony is achievable not because a group's individual members are all the same but because all individuals realise that each member is a reflective practitioner – taking account of the different members of the group and the environment in which it exists. Our lives all have different meanings – to deny this will result in rigidity and negativity – but taking the effort to integrate and link up different meanings we stand more chance of arriving at the brain's preferred state of harmony and coherence and to some extent the desired state of predictability.

So how can we help others to achieve a state of integration with their brain? The optimum emotional environment to help others with integration is one of compassion, understanding, sympathy, empathy and kindness. Under stress we are unlikely to be able to arrive at the calmer states of mind that assist the flow of integration.

Taking time to talk and listen to colleagues' stories and experiences about their lives, and taking an active decision to integrate, will help us all to survive mentally and emotionally within the workplace.

TAKING REGULAR TIME TO REFLECT

The brain is far happier when the outcomes of our behaviours and the behaviours of others are predictable. Predictable outcomes give more stability in our lives. The idea that we can rely on time for reflective practice creates an oasis in which the brain and mind can work together and integrate challenges – we begin to evolve as individuals and as a working group. For this reason it is important that we practise the evolving art of integration through the reflective practice time in our work or through any medium that gives a chance for further reflection.

Time out for reflective practice increases the functioning of our brain, helps us to grow our mind and will also increase our capacity to work through challenges as a group and our memberships of the larger whole. Ultimately as we transform our thinking, this leads to the act of transforming environments for the well-being of everyone – especially the service users who will feel understood because we have taken the time to understand ourselves in relationship with them.

The act of sitting quietly for 20 minutes a day with a focus on the question, 'How am I now?' will increase the art of mindfulness. For this you could keep a diary if that helps you and this would be an effective way to notice your development. I still have a diary that I kept on my mindfulness from 20 years ago.

Neuroscientists are now finding that the area of the brain known as the middle prefrontal cortex is the seat of the higher aspects of our self, housing the energy for key behaviour including: our ability to empathise, our body awareness, our intuition, our insight, emotion regulation including the ability to modulate fear, as well as our ability to attune to others.

In addition to this the middle prefrontal cortex is able to over-ride our cognitive mind by the ability to create a pause and wait for more information before we formulate a conclusion (Siegel 2010a). If we give ourselves a chance on a daily basis to allow this aspect of the brain to fire up and participate and integrate with other aspects of the brain, it can be seen that it is possible to increase our capacity to be more thoughtful and thus more mindful and ultimately more effective in our lives. None of this increase in our functioning you may notice relates in any way to buying more, having more or even going on expensive holidays. It is about giving yourself time to think. Time out and time to think develops the highest aspects of our functioning.

Once you have stopped your everyday mind from planning and predicting, you may have a sense of pausing and giving the mind time to breathe – as you in turn notice your breathing.

Try to remember that you can also engage in the art of imagination and creation as a way to inspire or even heal yourself or as a way in which to find relief from stress or difficulty. You can imagine and picture solutions that will give you solace 'for now' or even give you a new goal to work towards.

Try this simple exercise.

- Give yourself time to sit and reflect on how you are right now.

- As you sit you could notice the rhythm of your breathing in and out of your body.

- You could notice the state of your body. Where is the tension?

- As you notice tension you could tell those areas of the body 'relax' and they will. For example, tell your right shoulder to relax.

- This act of mindfulness may involve an act of assertion: asking people to give you 20 minutes while you sit quietly.

- Notice the quality of your thinking.

- What emotions are you experiencing – they may well be mixed.

- What is on your 'to do' list?

- What is on you 'what happens next' list?

- What is on your 'what do I plan to do once this is finished' list?

- How long does it take before you begin to settle?

- Are there any pictures or images that come to mind?

- And finally – can you give yourself a turbo charge boost towards the end of your mindfulness by imagining beautiful scenery or a scenario in which you are receiving a positive experience – like imagining you are bathing in sunlight, walking on a warm beach or floating in a calm Mediterranean sea?

CONCLUSION

In simple terms, mindfulness is the act of becoming more aware of how you work as an individual, becoming more familiar with your own regulatory style, your own anxieties and the thoughts that run through your mind. You actually have more control over your own states of mind than you think. It is likely that all of us will experience times when we feel we are out of control and that the limbic or emotional and affective seat of the mind has taken over, but if you are aware of exactly how you work you can manage your mind just as much as you please. The mind is such an effective piece of machinery that, if given a chance, it will regulate itself most effectively if it has been allowed to adopt this habit. Since our mind is also part of our relationships with others, mindfulness also involves thinking about our key relationships.

I am often concerned that the term mindfulness is one of those words that are thrown out without much understanding of what it really involves. Real mindfulness takes real action to make the brain work smoothly: it needs commitment, some time out of the 'doing' mode, support from others to take time out and just a little bit of hope.

SUMMARY

- Dan Siegel's definition of mind is useful to consider in relation to reflective practice, as it identifies the mind within ourselves, but also in our relationships with others (Siegel 2010a).

- The brain and mind work best in positive emotional environments. Children's brains are open to learning in positive emotional states such as joy, but children are frightened by negative responses and may become closed to learning.

- The brain has the potential to flow freely, but also the potential on the one hand to become caught in rigidity or on the other hand lost in chaos.

- Siegel describes the flow of the brain as having five aspects – Flexibility, Adaptability, Coherence, Energy and Stability which help us to see the potential of the brain to be flexible and adaptive to change (Siegel 2010a).

- We may engage in unconscious behaviours that bring balance and harmony in our daily lives. These could be behaviours such as smoking, daydreaming, or drinking tea (although smoking will be a health hazard and you may wish to notice how you use smoking time when in fact you are really trying to be more mindful).

- A mindfulness exercise might include writing down your thoughts, focusing the mind on an object or noticing your breathing or just taking some time out.

- The brain integrates all the information it receives into a coherent whole. If we take this theory and put it at the centre of our practice with children, we start to see that we are helping children to integrate various aspects of themselves such as emotional, cognitive, memory, body, relational.

- It's beneficial to take regular opportunities to reflect.

- In our imagination we can create and heal ourselves and we can paint our future – reflection can be creative too.

Chapter 4

STEPPING STONES TO REFLECTIVE PRACTICE
THINKING TOOLS

People may choose not to adopt a reflective stance, because they have not been persuaded that it is helpful to them. They may not have been given the tools and footholds into reflective practice. This chapter is designed to introduce you to some further ideas which you can use when engaging in reflective and mindful practice.

BLOCKED THINKING

I observe many parents and carers who fail to think about things simply because they do not know or have forgotten *how* to think about things. Caring for children is intense work, and adults can become stuck in familiar routines, and feel tired or despondent. Often adults can mirror their child's state – children will often engage in difficult behaviours because their minds are stuck in a state of despair if they have no support for their problems and no one can help them out.

Imagine how hard it must be for a young child when all they are able to do is act out their problem through their behaviour, only to find that the person with whom they are trying to communicate reacts in an unhelpful way. This is the beginning of a process of despair.

In fact children can become so psychologically distressed that when they cannot express their anxiety or fear to a relevant adult they start to use illness as a way to cope with the emotional pain that they experience with 'somatoform' disorders or hypochondriacal disorders where psychological symptoms are expressed through concern over the body. The body therefore is a mirror of the state of their mind.

I should stress that I am not suggesting that illness in children is due to psychological difficulties in any way at all. There are, however, some somatic complaints that children endure that are highly likely to be linked to their state of mind (ICD-10 1993, and DSM-IV 2000). This is often happening when we see children who are physically lethargic and unable to move and enjoy action. Frequently such children are terrified to move. It is often the case that children who cannot process psychological material through the supportive mind of an adult and in relationship with carers, actually start to experience psychosomatic symptoms such as digestive problems, bowel problems and stomach aches (again I am talking about somatic symptoms and not real illness in a child). We also see disorders such elective mutism (choosing not to speak), non-organic enuresis (wetting) and non-organic encopresis (soiling) (ICD-10 1993).

The digestive system could be seen as a metaphor for processing and eliminating matter through the body – just as the brain processes mental matter through the mind. Through reflection the brain successfully resolves problems and sees them through to a state of equilibrium. The body does the same, processing and digesting food through to a state of elimination and equilibrium. Children with psychological problems which are not addressed frequently experience parallel problems with elimination such as enuresis and encopresis (wetting and soiling) as mentioned above. Details of this can be found in The World Health Organization's classification of Mental and Behavioural Disorders (ICD-10 1993).

Several years ago I observed a child who had been chronically constipated for five years receive psychological support from her new carer. Aided by some thoughtful support from a foster parent who was mindful of her difficulties, combined with some medication from an equally thoughtful doctor, the child overcame her chronic elimination problem in a matter of six weeks. Not only did she cease to live in pain, she also started to digest food properly, regained her appetite and began to grow properly. The chronic 'stuckness' within her mind and system had actually reduced her appetite so that she was no longer growing and was underweight and undersized for her six years of age. This was a girl who came from an environment in which her emotional life was ignored and her fears particularly were dismissed.

It is possible for the same blocked level of thinking and poor emotional literacy to occur in childcare scenarios and it is not hard to see how. Frequently it occurs because staff teams around a child engage in their own closed culture and they are not given the tools to get out of their own familiar thinking patterns.

This is the same for cultures within any organisation, but people offering a service to those who are vulnerable without the capacity to reflect on experience is equivalent to a culture which defends itself from the needs of those who are vulnerable. If that culture stays the same without change, it simply becomes dysfunctional and caters primarily for its own needs.

SHIFTING BLOCKED THINKING: A CASE EXAMPLE

A lot of work with complex cases with children requires a shift in thinking, a change of perspective or an adjustment of mindset. As an example I have used a piece of transformative work undertaken with a team in Europe with a teenager in care who wished to change sexual identity.

He was a robust and muscular young man and it seemed so unlikely that he would wish to change gender and become a young woman. When he first began talking about this his team completely dismissed his ideas and his attempts to communicate with them about it. They laughed at him in a jovial way trying to tease him out of his new plan. They were not unkind, but they just could not conceptualise or get close to his motivation to change and of course their response to him was hurtful – despite the fact that they had not intended this. They just could not take him seriously. The young man became very restless and challenging as it became clear to him that people were not going to take him seriously. He lost his connection with his team and his care became fragmented, and interactions with the carers were filled with painful aggression. The team reacted defensively and they felt lost in their work with him.

In reflective practice the team allowed themselves to sit with the idea that this young man might have meant what he was saying to them. As they let this idea seep into their minds, they began to feel quite sad and understand how isolated he must feel in this process. They began to explore ways that they could invite him again to consider sharing his process with them (as he had been trying to do). They thought about ways that they could regain his trust and engage in dialogue.

They also explored in an open and honest way their prejudice against transgender men – the team were mostly all male. They reflected on their nervousness about this, how they did not understand the basis for it, and how it threatened their world view of gender orientation. Their only real knowledge of transgender experience was through bad jokes and funny films. There was some laughter about transgender exploration between them, but when this quietened down it turned into sadness about their dismissiveness of the young man in their care and the loss of relationship with him.

They wondered what it might feel like to be so misunderstood at such an early age. Once they had travelled through this process together they then began planning for a new future and a new environment for him. One member of the team apologised on behalf of them all for not understanding, and another gathered information from transgender websites. One man even went shopping with their client to second-hand shops to buy clothes and consider clothing options, and through this the real work began with their young client whom they now saw as vulnerable rather than ridiculous. He also no longer threatened their view of the world.

In another reflective practice session they were able to discuss the view that they could hear what the young person was saying, but that they secretly hoped he would change his mind. Nonetheless, they had re-established the connection and relationship with the young person, the aggression had settled, and they were having cheerful experiences together. In later sessions the team fully accepted that the young person would be changing from male to female and they supported him in this process. The team were fully behind him to the point that they defended him from as many difficulties and prejudices as possible that emerged in his life. Many of them pointed out that they would never have thought that their thinking could shift so effectively from one position to another.

IMPROVING REFLECTIVE FUNCTIONING

How do we get better at reflective functioning? Peter Fonagy has been working with Mary Target at University College London for some years on the concept of 'reflective functioning'. He describes this as, 'The ability to give meaning to mental states of others as well as ourselves by the explanations that we attribute to our experience' (Fonagy and Target 1997, p.679). In other words it helps us to make sense of and understand ourselves and others. This can be seen as an organic functioning of the brain to organise material into meaningful states of mind. He refers directly to the ability to distinguish between our inner and outer lives, to make sense of mental and emotional processes and to be able to reflect both on our own experience as well as our interpersonal experiences with others. It could be seen as a way to organise experience and make sense of it as well as a way to regulate ourselves.

Throughout the rest of the chapter, I describe some of the other key ideas and theories which can be used to understand reflective practice and its potential – the 'building blocks' for reflective practice which can help us to see how a reflective environment can be developed to help people.

INNER LIFE AND OUTER LIFE

To understand effective communication and increased reflective capacity, we need to be able to take on board the basic premise that human beings have both an inner life and an outer life. Their outer life may relate to the things that they do and the things that they have to do – their behaviours. An inner life relates to the world of our thoughts, feelings and emotions, all of which we can hide from others if we wish or communicate to others if we wish. We are the gatekeepers to our own privacy. Our inner world of thoughts or feelings is our very own private world. By the age of seven children are quite capable of being aware of their inner and outer lives. They can name basic emotions and talk about their feelings and they will be aware that their actions may not be the same as what goes on inside them. For example, they are able to cover up a feeling if they are upset at school which they may express later when they get home. It would seem that human beings have developed this capacity in order to survive socially. If a child is upset at school they realise that it is not quite the same as getting really upset and angry at home and that their emotions may not be tolerated or understood in the same way as in their home (although I have noted with some children that the reverse is true). They might understand quite instinctively that they need to 'put on a little more face' in school.

If we are going to think about thinking – which is what we do in reflective practice – we will be taking time to link up our inner world of thoughts and feelings and our outer world of actions and events so that we are more congruent with both aspects of ourselves. In the process of accepting this basic premise of the human mind, we give ourselves the chance to integrate and bring together two separate aspects of our brain – the doing brain and the being brain.

In acknowledging this basic complexity of your mind, it's possible to start to notice more about how you respond in the world; to notice things like how much tension you deal with in the course of your day, how many different things you need to think about at one moment in time, and how very busy and demanding your life might be. Just sitting and noticing these things is very productive, despite the fact that it appears to be a passive act. To sit and notice what you feel inside and what you have been doing is a beginning to reflective practice.

To sit with others and notice what they are thinking and feeling will also tell you about yourself as you resonate and respond to them. That is an act of group reflective practice.

ATTUNEMENT

Dan Siegel refers to this as the way in which we focus on the flow of information and energy when we are relating to others in an 'open and receptive manner' (Siegel 2012a, p.23).

However, the term became common language following the work of Dan Stern in 1998 when he was writing about parental care of infants and their capacity to care for that infant through attunement. He felt that attunement was an optimum activity to be engaged in with a baby in order to develop the attachment relationship to a secure degree (Stern 1998).

Attunement is when we stop ourselves for a moment in order to give ourselves a chance to understand more deeply the energetic exchange that is taking place between two people. We soften our need to interact quickly or to impress others and take control and we give ourselves a moment of calm just as we might do if we were approaching a newborn child. As we do this we start to take note of aspects of the person engaged in the communication such as the signals that they have on their face that are there for us to read and we 'tune in' to those signals. As we soften to others and use our senses we are able to take in more information about them. If we are softer and more sensitive to ourselves we may find better solutions to our own everyday problems and we may be more compassionate and less judgemental. In attuning to the children we work with, we are giving them a better standard of attention. As a result they may be more soothed and more comfortable. Attention is vital nourishment for children and adults. Attunement is the right kind of attention at the right time.

SENSITIVITY

Sensitivity means that we are aware of the needs of both ourselves and others and that we respond to them accurately and as soon as we can. There is no sensitivity if we listen to the needs of a client or patient or child and then push what they have said out of our minds.

Sensitivity requires some effective response to show that we are engaging in the well-being of the other. We can be sensitive to others, but totally insensitive to ourselves and our own needs. This is not necessarily a good idea and ultimately leads to carer burnout. Just as in flight safety before an aeroplane takes off, we are reminded of the need to put on our own oxygen mask in order that we can assist our neighbour with theirs, we need to take care of our own needs first.

THEORY OF MIND: ACKNOWLEDGING DIFFERENT MINDS AND PERSPECTIVES

'Theory of Mind' is a theory proposed by the researcher Flavell (Flavell 1999). According to Flavell we reach a developmental stage at around the age of four as a pre-schooler when we realise that the whole world does not revolve around our mind, and that we are not all thinking the same thing. There is not an exact age for achieving the developmental goal of having a 'Theory of Mind'. Some children might achieve it slightly earlier than others, especially if they have a large sibling group and they are constantly observing their interactions, but it is not a mark of higher IQ – more a marker of practice in social interactions. Essentially children start to overcome the egocentricity (the idea that the world revolves around the individual) of their toddler life. Children start to acknowledge that others may have viewpoints that are different from their own. This is the beginning of the capacity to understand the intentions of others which is a skill that enhances communication and on the whole eases distress in communication.

On the whole the Theory of Mind leads a pre-schooler to innately understand that minds exist, that they are not concrete objects, but they enable us to represent and interpret our experience and the experience of others. Children of course will not be able to quote this theory to you – it is an innate awareness that develops particularly as the child is socialising. It is a flow of energy through the brain that is asking, 'What is going on around me?' This question could be vital to survival.

IMAGINATION AND THE BRAIN

Pre-school children begin to realise that there can be a difference between what they think and what they see and that which is actually true. So they begin to engage in 'pretend play' – they may pretend to be a policeman or a burglar; they know that they are not in reality. A friend may come along and say, 'I am a monster.' The pre-schooler can see very clearly that there is no monster, but he or she may engage in a terrifying and thrilling game of monsters just the same. This is imaginary play. As soon as pre-school children develop the capacity to do it, they love to engage in pretending, and it is great fun for them, but they know it is not real.

Children can use pretend play to both enjoy themselves and act out emerging ideas about their world – they can also resolve anxieties through pretend play and demonstrate their feelings. So, for example, a child cuddling a dolly and being a mummy may also be giving themselves comfort or showing us what they need and like. One child who I worked with nursed a doll for many sessions, but would not let me talk about his own need to be nursed. It did not matter, because it gave him peace of mind and a sense of calm, because in his imagination he was providing a healing experience. This remarkable development in the mind becomes the imagination of the adult mind in which we can create new worlds if we wish that are different from our reality – and our imagination can be the source of innovation for science and culture as well as healing and art.

Paul Gilbert in *The Compassionate Mind* (Gilbert 2010) refers to the development of the 'new brain' and describes imagination as part of our brain's evolution whereby we can be fully aware of reality and at the same time create new worlds. By referring to 'new brain' he is referring to the most sophisticated and creative aspect of the brain as opposed to the more primitive aspects of the brain (the limbic system) that were developed millions of years before the new brain.

Gilbert (2010) notes that with our new brain we can imagine and we can also make plans for the future and anticipate and make predictions about what we will do. He explains how our imagination can be both a source of power and development, but it can also be a source of fear and debilitation or even illness in that as much as we can imagine wonderful creations we can also imagine terrible things. The problem being that part of our brain – the limbic system, which he refers to as 'old brain', starts to think that what we imagine is real and will react accordingly by sending out hormones to respond to the imagined problem.

If you have a deep anxiety that your house may be broken into and that you will be robbed, you can easily convince your brain that this is actually happening and the brain will react to defend you. You alert your limbic system to expect trouble. Equally if you use your imagination to create pictures of wonderful solutions and soothing experiences – including thoughts of compassion and kindness towards yourself – you are likely to convince your limbic system that all is well and you can reduce stress. If you imagine you are walking on a sandy beach with the sun shining your whole body will begin to respond accordingly. However, we must face reality here. If it is likely that your house is going to be broken into you need to do something about securing your home rather than sitting in fear – there is no point in imagining a nice sandy beach as the robbers sneak by with a swag bag.

So, whilst our imagination is a rich source of creativity and healing, we have to manage its power over the brain. Mindfulness can be a most useful tool for tracking and keeping us aware of our imagination and how it may be affecting our brain's behaviour. In a similar way it can be used to help children recognise their own imaginations and to enable them to use their minds to create calm solutions.

Since so much of young people's worlds might be tied up in receiving information that is violent, aggressive and frightening through visual images, such as from TV and computer games, it's worth reflecting on the effect this has on their limbic system leaving them ready to 'fight'. A child may be fed lots of materialistic or aggressive information through a computer game which creates expectations about what they can do in the world.

In the real and relational world we are restricted in what we can do by relational and social codes, but children who have not had supportive parenting to develop their capacity to control their own limbic system often have difficulty in understanding or integrating this experience. We wonder why we have so many children who are more aggressive and out of control. It is the task of adult carers to help children to understand and learn new ways to control their reactive primitive systems, and to be able to do that the adult needs to lead by example; to show the skills children need to develop and provide an environment in which they can value the rewards of self-management and self-control.

The beauty of the imagination is the fact that it is so powerful and creative. Whilst you can choose to use your time spent reflecting to concentrate on reality, it can also be used to image desirable solutions and outcomes. Of course it is possible to get carried away, but this capacity of the mind is what is going to move things forward. If we cannot imagine a solution, we may remain stuck where we are.

CHANGING YOUR MIND

Human beings benefit from the ability to change our minds, and we have evolved a fluid capacity to rethink and engage in new behaviours: reflective practice at its best.

Psychiatrist and neurobiologist Dan Siegel refers to a range of states between rigid and controlled on the one hand, and flexible and potentially chaotic on the other hand (Siegel 2010a). An extreme of either state is undesirable and probably needs some attention and management: chaos and lack of control means that a person is not managing the flow of their mind, while excess rigidity means that they are over-controlling the flow of information and energy.

In fact Siegel (2010a) proposes that it may be possible for psychiatrists to write a manual of mental illness or well-being based on this range of states where excess rigidity of the mind could be referred to as depression and total chaos of the mind could be referred to as hypermania. Somewhere in the middle, when the mind is functioning with a good flow of energy, we have the ability to alter our mind states, or given the right conditions they may even alter themselves.

So, a bad mood at the start of the day based on a preoccupying worry may clear into a cheerful state by lunch time.

A state of upset over some event may last for a few hours or even a few days, or in the case of grief at the loss of a loved one perhaps a few years, but that state will move on into a newly formed picture and a new set of values or goals with our memory holding and protecting our picture of the loved one we once knew.

Ultimately it works very much for us as human beings that we can quite literally change our mind, and that in changing our mind our brain will be shifting and integrating new information and energy.

Changing minds also happens on a larger scale. For example, consensus opinions relating to homosexuality, equality, race and health issues have changed radically over decades past as people are exposed to new information and changed environments, but often this change is initiated by an individual or small group and their courage to reflect on events and admit that they have changed their mind.

As well as having the ability to change our minds, we also have the ability to change our judgement. Neuroscience has found that the mind is made to be judgemental about the things that it senses so that it can scrutinise whether they are useful to survival; however, we can be more aware of the quality of the judgements that we are making.

A judgement could be helpful and give useful information, or it could be denigrating and abusive. The most effective mindful people are those who are aware that their judgements move on with time. They do not become concrete about their thinking or over-identified with the moment-by-moment judgements that they have to make.

To apply this principle of the value of flexibility to work with children, your practice needs to take place in an environment in which you can change your mind or even be in two minds about something. I have a much-practised phrase, 'I have been thinking about that…and I have to let you know that I changed my mind.' We need to be aware of how easily we can slip into a mindset or fixed way of thinking as a group and forget to welcome new ideas into that group. There are dire examples throughout the history of group thinking that force out new ideas or 'questions' about the group. Here is one very dire example relating to childcare from which we all need to learn.

CASE EXAMPLE: ABUSE IN A DAY NURSERY

In 2009, a day nursery was closed down when it was finally realised that up to 30 children, including infants under the age of one, had been sexually molested by a female paedophile working in the nursery on a daily basis.

The critical case review by the Local Safeguarding Authority revealed that the staff team had uncomfortable feelings for months about the member of staff concerned, including awareness of her sexualised language and inappropriate pornography on her mobile phone.

Everyone indicated that they felt uncomfortable about this. The perpetrator was a forceful personality and she was also quite a social character – rather fun to be with and very much a leader in the group on a social level; she also tended to be 'in' with the team manager. Not one person felt able to raise concerns about her behaviour despite the fact that in their mind they had concerns. There was poor supervision and there was not a healthy environment to raise questions or concerns. There was certainly no opportunity to think clearly outside of the daily culture of the nursery.

Clearly this is an extreme example of an environment in which the capacity to think and reflect has been pushed to the back of the agenda, and I know that people who care for children (including myself) are likely to feel uncomfortable reflecting on this – but the issue has to be raised – how bad can it get when people refuse to use their minds and reflect on experience?

The answer is that it can get really bad: without reflection life degenerates into unprocessed behaviours without any real meaning.

With reflective practice we can reach the heights of our capability to be creative and think out of the box – we can also do the very important work of housekeeping, cleaning up the problems, and facing down the difficulties so that we have a mindful and secure base for the creativity that we can achieve.

BEING CONCERNED WITH OTHERS

The idea that we are innately programmed to be concerned with others, so that we understand how they are thinking, is an exciting idea for the layperson and neuroscientist alike (Schore 1994). Babies are born with an innate openness to discover what is in a face: they look to the face of their carers and are entranced by what they see, studying faces intently in their quiet private moments, and become 'little professors' of understanding the expressions and changes in the faces that they study.

Through the act of studying faces, babies discover which faces make them feel good and which they do not want to see. By the time a baby is six months old, they have quite clear ideas about their preferences with regard to people and, of course, as we have discovered above, by the time they are pre-schoolers they start to have a growing knowledge of how minds work and how they can read minds through reading faces.

Although this behaviour turns out to be a key to social skill, it begins as a key to safety and survival – as do most behaviours in infants. The child seeks to predict the intentions or thoughts of the adults who care for them so that they can insure that someone is there to meet their needs. If those adults are more predictable the child will be less anxious about this. If those adults are less predictable and more chaotic, the child will be more anxious about this and constantly monitor the adult for their intentions.

As reflective practitioners it is crucial that we are aware of these underlying aspects of human behaviour so that we interpret children's behaviour accurately and respond sensitively.

DEVELOPMENTAL STAGES: WORKING WITH THE CHILDREN AS INDIVIDUALS

A common mistake made when caring for vulnerable children is to fail to take into account the developmental stage of the child.

If a carer tells me, 'I spent a long time arguing with the six-year-old,' I know immediately that they need some more information about the developmental state of a six-year-old and some reflective practice on what it is like to be six.

Sometimes children can be placed under a great deal of stress when adults assume that they have the same mind as an adult, and forget that they are children. In order to be smart in our reflective practice or functioning it is important to remember this.

Similarly, if you are working with a young adult who has Down's syndrome, you need to allow for the challenges that she has in information processing – she will be slightly slower to make sense of information and may need more time and support.

The key point is to take difference into consideration.

Reflect on your own life: as a young child, you may have thought about a subject in one way, then as a teenager from a different perspective, and then as an adult from yet another perspective. For example, a five-year-old may idealise her parents, but that same child as a teenager may denigrate her parents. That same teenager as an adult may have a realistic appraisal of her parents and may accept them as they are. All of these behaviours would be age appropriate and Mums and Dads and carers have to be able to withstand these developmental changes in children from infancy to adulthood.

The mind's view changes as a result of developmental leaps, and changes in its ability to process information.

RECIPROCAL COMMUNICATION

We rely heavily on each other for our very existence – something which may be forgotten in societies where individuality is prized. There is an interdependence at every level of society.

Take the simple example of an aircraft taking off. It takes hundreds of different people doing very different jobs to get that aircraft cruising – from the person who checks in the luggage to the pilot, the engineer, the cleaner, and staff responsible for air traffic control, keeping the tarmac clear, making sure the doors are closed and making the meals. There is a network of interdependent activity involved, and if the group responsible is not of one mind in its actions, then there could be a problem.

In the same way, if carers are not of one mind and do not share the flow of information and energy that childcare involves, then critical incidents can result or at the least the child is very confused. Individual members in any group need to be able to link their thinking and activities just as the aircraft operational group have one goal in mind – to get the aircraft safely in the air. The care group need to share information and energy in order to allow the child to experience an optimum environment that cares for them.

This is reciprocity: social glue which serves as the basis of all communication and interpersonal interaction. The capacity for reciprocity begins in infancy and proceeds throughout our lives. Parents give children their first experience of reciprocal relationships by caring for them sensitively and children 'internalise' this model of experience, in turn using it as their own model. Children learn to dance with others in the style of 'give and take'. If children are starved of reciprocity in early childhood, they are deeply affected, but the brain remains open and has a certain amount of plasticity to allow for a chance for change (Schore 1994).

Children may well learn more about reciprocity as they grow older from their friends, partners and colleagues and engage in contented social interactions. At school children learn to play one another's games; they share and find mutuality.

Reflective practice provides another learning opportunity where the detail of our interactions can be analysed. Reciprocity is the capacity to work in step with each other, and sadly many children who have been neglected or abused by parental care will not have developed this art, but this does not mean that they do not want it, or are not able to find it.

It is the 'give and take' of relationships in life that most people take for granted when it is working; when it fails, a common response is to be upset or alarmed, and to instinctively attempt to make good a relationship.

It takes courage to work with children who are not reciprocal in relationships, and beyond courage it takes much thought and planning. How do you plan your interaction with a child to help them to relate more effectively? How can you help a child to give something back so that they get a 'feel' for giving when they consistently shut you out and make caring for them unrewarding? This is a very difficult scenario to tolerate unless we are understanding of why that behaviour exists.

These are extremely useful things to consider during reflective practice sessions. You may even be able to help a child reflect on their own actions and notice for themselves what they think they need to give.

DOING REFLECTIVE PRACTICE IN THE WORKPLACE

It's common for an initial response to being asked to engage in reflective practice to be defensive: staff may feel disgruntled about having to look further into things when they are already working so hard.

I recall one of my students referring to one of my art work reflective practice sessions as 'psychobabble rubbish'. I was not actually offended by this as I could see the point she was trying to make, because maybe using another part of the brain to think may have felt a bit like taking a mind altering drug. Later this same young woman wrote me a letter and apologised saying that she was having a stressful time in her life and that her work was very demanding and causing her some pain – she felt angry that her organisation was not supporting her.

Through this information sharing process we were able to engage in a compassionate and meaningful discussion about where help was needed and what could be done to put things right. This turned out to be a marvellously productive act of reflection, integration and understanding for us both in which all of the issues came to the surface and became well-organised. The previously dammed up anxiety and stress in the mind actually became a flow of information and energy that said, 'Things are not right for me.' A moment of resistance and anger often arises like this just before people are going to let that flow of information and energy happen, and it can be frightening and unnerving especially if they work in an environment where they are unused to the luxury of being allowed to be 'open'. The woman concerned was just about to have to say that her organisation was not supporting her to do the right thing – that was a big and frightening thing to be saying. But it was also the truth and the truth actually matters in reflective practice.

The question is – do we want an open and communicative flow of information and energy between us as an organisation in which our minds can function at their best, or do we want our minds to be closed and dammed up? This creates a rather murky and potentially dangerous psychological environment in which our brains and organisations become closed down nobody moves forward, and we are potentially harmful and not helpful to the people we are supposed to support. I might add that through that scenario I became even more determined to present mindfulness practice and reflective practice in ways that could not be construed as 'strange' but more as 'sensible'. So that was a powerful piece of learning for me too.

Caring for children who are vulnerable is difficult and complicated work, and can take its toll on the mindset of individuals and teams. However, it is extremely damaging when a team of workers adopt a negative outlook: it can lead to negative behaviours such as malicious gossip, collusion and scapegoating.

In my experience, such behaviours can be symptoms of depressive tendencies in the team and will lead to a degeneration of skill. It may occur when a team has been pushed to its limits, perhaps caring for children who are acting out aggressively and violently or abusively. If abusive exchanges continue, I have witnessed teams becoming despondent and despairing and acting out the level of abuse they have experienced. Children are then dragged into a quagmire of unconscious and negative exchanges.

Vulnerable children are harmed by this additional pressure in their lives, especially considering that their experiences to date are likely to have been a 'toxic soup' of unprocessed emotions and passive aggression towards them. Carers need to be very clear that children cannot help this – it is part of their condition.

This is not to say that negative emotions should be banned. We all have them, and in some sense they are a powerful communication to us to say that we are on the edge of our coping skills and feel hopeless about our survival, or that we simply need to pay attention to something that is happening. We must face our negative experiences and reactions and try to fully understand them rather than turning our backs and pretending they are not happening.

Reflective practice is needed to create a more constructive and conscious environment in which there are rewards for organising mental and emotional material. The greatest reward of all is that a team should engage in more positive states of mind with more positive emotions, and that negative states should be soothed and calmed with healthy solutions to problems.

SUMMARY

In this chapter I have underlined why it is important to engage in reflective practice when we are faced with complicated states in children which need to be unravelled by mindful carers. I have also underlined some of the building blocks which enable us to understand the nature and potential of reflective practice.

- Theory provides us with the 'building blocks' to understanding children and practise effective reflection.

- The theory and ideas covered in this chapter provide us with an opportunity to think about how we can employ reflection to the best advantage of children in our care.

- Be open to the positive potential of changing your mind.

- Children are innately concerned with others.

- Don't make assumptions based on children's developmental ages.

- Reflect on the potential of reciprocal relationships.

- As well as the potential positive uses of reflective practice, it plays a critical part in avoiding critical incidents and negative workplace culture.

Chapter 5

YOUR STORY MATTERS

It is important to understand that people bring their individual stories with them both in their personality and behaviours.

LIFE STORIES AND BELIEF SYSTEMS

We are our life stories. Our individual life stories influence our thinking and behaviour. In short our own personal history and our memories are our own personal psychology. People are all psychologists at heart – trying to make sense of experiences, and anticipating and wondering about the intentions and experiences of others. We are born to have an autobiography inside us, stored in our memories as a unique story of our own. If practitioners wish to work effectively with children and young people, a very good starting point is to become more aware of their own tendencies and then to become aware of the influence these tendencies may have on a young person's life. As a practitioner considers their own individual story, they will become more authentic with helping young people consider the impact of life events on their own lives. This is the most basic form of psychological awareness that answers the fundamental question that many young people carry with them – who am I?

Ultimately you have become your history and you cannot change that. Whether a child's story is painful, privileged, diverse, abusive, exciting or boring – it's all their very own piece of the world. The first step to more personal awareness and freedom of thinking is to be able to accept that story and all that it reveals about how you have become a person. As a result of reflecting on your story, you may start to notice life patterns and you may want to correct any negative tendencies or rethink some life strategies. Bowlby has said:

> The therapist's task is to enable his patient to recognize that his (her) images of him/herself and of others, derived either from past painful experiences or from misleading messages emanating from a parent…may or may not be appropriate to his present and future or indeed may never have been justified. (Bowlby 1988, p.157)

On the other hand you may bring some brilliant ideas with you from your life story. We inherit productive and positive values too. Essentially we internalise our experience and it feeds the ground of our inherited value system (the ground being our mind). We have already used a common example of a value system about children – 'if they misbehave they are naughty'. What if your life story has led you to believe that children who behaved badly are just naughty? This may come about because rather than understand your behaviour as a child your parents (or carers) just reacted to you from their inherited belief that if children are not good then they are naughty.

If your behaviour was inconvenient or unusual they may have referred to you as bad – or they are very likely to have misinterpreted your intentions, failing to recognise and take into consideration your stage of development or the vulnerability of the immature mind. That is a commonly held belief in our society today and understandable although particularly unhelpful especially to children. For example, I have observed plenty of two-year-olds referred to as 'naughty' by parents who simply do not understand the developmental stage of a two-year-old. If they were able to consider and reflect on the behaviour of the average two-year-old, they would accept exploration and tantrums as the wonderful roots and beginnings of self-assertion and deal with it compassionately. I observed one adult parent refer to their two-year-old as having 'an anger management problem'. In fact they were just having a normal and very healthy tantrum.

It is not possible that children are just bad with a desire to be naughty, even if our own emotional instincts might tell us otherwise. In fact all behaviour in children is an effort to communicate and relate in order to stay safe combined with an impulse to explore their environment and discover. If you are alive it is almost imperative to respond to the internal impulse to communicate (unless of course we are poorly or depressed or suffering in some way) and our brains urge us to discover new things. In really it is far more likely that children naturally love to co-operate and lead a happy and productive life. They just need to be supported and moved in this direction. More often than not if children are difficult they are anxious or sad or maybe even mad and angry – but rarely just bad.

REFLECT ON YOUR STORY

Take the time to step back and reflect. If you are arguing with a child (I mean any child, toddler to teenager) you are doing the wrong thing. If you are understanding or at least making attempts to understand a child's behaviour you are probably doing the right thing. Why would you argue with a child who is half your size and half your brain capacity? Arguing with a child because they are believed to be naughty is a simple example of a value system that needs to shift in order to help young people – rather than make them even more angry and disappointed in adults. But it takes time to step back and reflect on how a child is behaving and it takes some confidence in the process of being reflective.

The more you reflect and formulate healthier conclusions, the more that process brings results and works effectively, and the more that you are able to gain a reflexive awareness of your life story in its influence on you – it may have led you to have a belief system that is unhelpful and you can overcome this by taking time to think.

In my research and work with young people and carers, I have found that the combination of self-awareness combined with excellent training in reflective practice gives a secure base to our thinking consisting of the most important ingredient that we can find – our capacity to reflect on and understand more deeply the needs of the young person in our care (North 2010).

Below, I model this behaviour using some personal narratives and stories – each one of us has a story which is unique and personal, and it is who we have become. This idea of a life story is reflected in psychotherapy and in attachment theory (Bowlby 1988) when we ask about a person's history or their attachment experience. The question is asked not out of curiosity, but because your personality will be the sum total of your story – whether it's a tough story or not – and you have to own your own history and understanding of the past in order to aim for the story that you want in the future.

CHILDREN CLAIMING THEIR STORY

Children and young people have stories – their history – their experience, and it's desirable to encourage them to claim the fabric of their story so that they can make sense of it and move on if necessary.

This process needs to be age and case appropriate of course. We can only expect children to claim as much as possible of their story, and children may omit certain experiences behind them such as trauma or things that have caused excessive shame. That has to be respected.

However, as a general rule practitioners cannot expect children to do what we ourselves do not do. If children see that you represent a coherent and well-managed person with acceptance of your own inner life – as far as possible making sense of your thoughts and feelings and impulses – they will copy and 'internalise' that behaviour. Human beings love to mimic the behaviour that they see.

Practitioners will not necessarily be telling the children they work with their own story, but children will see very quickly and notice whether or not carers are comfortable and accepting of who they are, so that they might learn ways to be comfortable and accepting of themselves.

This process can be especially difficult if children are suffering from trauma and have complex and traumatic stories. Children should not ever be forced to remember their story; instead it should be a gradual journey of learning for the child. My proposal is that children will learn better self-acceptance and better psychological skills if the adult caring for them is able to model those very basic skills and has themself found security in their own life.

MY OWN STORY

I don't expect people to do what I won't do, so this chapter continues by exploring by way of illustration some aspects of my own personal story which led to my own sense of self.

There has been much learning in my life over the last 17 years, starting with the day that I worked at a school for children with emotional and behavioural disturbance.

The challenging child

A child one day was on a roof throwing rocks at staff and when one of those rocks was a near miss just past my head it certainly made me sit down and reflect on my role and how I could help this child – who might have just nearly killed me or at least caused some damage, because to me this child not only seemed out of control but lost to the minds who should be helping him – including my own.

Following the rock hurling the same child set fire to something in the yard that created so much toxic smoke (I think it was plastic) that I had to sit in my office for an hour before it was safe to be released. Now that certainly gained my attention. The whole school was in lockdown due to the toxic cloud that had been created by a very distressed young person. Nobody was harmed, but we were all wondering what this child was doing; the child had achieved his goal of bringing attention to himself which helped to heal his own isolation and perhaps give him a sense that others were concerned. I realised that I had no tools to understand him or his behaviour or even to help me feel compassionate towards him. If I could not find those tools, then I had better change my job because I did not have too much patience for near death experiences either from falling rocks or smoke inhalation and noxious fumes.

I gave myself a year to complete some of my learning towards this goal – of better understanding and more compassion for children with challenging behaviour before changing tack and taking up a different career. It was that moment of decision that led me to study in detail the principles of attachment theory and the way that it highlights the development of both personality and psychopathology in human beings.

Whilst attachment theory is not all of the answer to behavioural problems and there are many schools of thought we can draw on in order to help children – it is without doubt one of the most significant contributors to our understanding of the development of the human personality and behaviour arising in the last millennium.

My own challenging childhood

My desire to understand children in difficulty was driven by my own innate desire for safety and security for myself, my own children and for others. Attachment theory also helped me to understand my own drive or compulsion to ensure that environments are safe. Briefly, John Bowlby (1988) demonstrated that infant behaviours are aimed at optimum survival and that infants are primed to reach out to carers for a response to their vulnerability and helplessness. These behaviours – the way that we are constantly interacting in order to survive and develop are built into our nervous system and are the basis for our impulses in life. In short the way we are cared for is who we will become – with experience encoded into our autobiographical memory – always influencing how we think and the way that we behave.

With regard to my own compulsion for safety, it was not that I was raised in a particularly dangerous environment – I cannot say that it was an environment that easily left me feeling joyful – more that I had a responsibility to care for others.

There were certainly some interesting challenges that I faced when I was a child that perhaps geared me towards wanting to provide the right kind of environment for my own children to develop and learn. One of these challenges was the constant changes in school. In total I would have been registered at 11 schools between the age of 5 and 16…for the non-mathematicians among you – that did work out at one per year.

That is rather a lot and might suggest that nobody was in charge of my education or actually had their eye on the ball or any authority or control over what was happening. Education was in fact given low status in my family environment. I don't blame my parents for this because they were in fact victims of their own set of circumstances – in many senses they were economic migrants – moving from one place to another in order to maximise their income and life chances – including twice to Africa and many parts of the United Kingdom. In their struggle to survive – the importance of my education and that of my siblings was apparently lost to them – as far as they were concerned it was just another school they had to find for their children in another country as soon as possible.

As I reflect on their behaviour I can now understand some of the anxiety about economic survival that would have driven their own behaviour to the extent that they became blind to other aspects of survival that were less important to them – for example, neither of them had a formal secondary education beyond the age of 14. As far as I was concerned in my childhood, another school was yet another culture to which I had to adapt, quickly before I got moved on again. No wonder I grew up with the constant sense that I was an outsider and with a constant anxiety about my own levels of knowledge – about everything. However, whilst I should not exaggerate the impact of this educationally challenging experience, this was not the worst kind of challenge and, as is often the case, those kinds of disadvantage make people struggle to achieve far greater things than they have experienced.

My parents would never have understood that in their desperate struggle for economic equality – they actually violated my right to learn and made me struggle for stability. The fact that I have achieved a master's degree and a doctorate in my subject is probably more due to the sense of loss of education in my childhood as to the need to prove my ability. Most people don't usually have to gain a doctorate in order to prove themselves. So perhaps those tough conditions have propelled me forward. It has certainly made me passionate about the possibility of learning from everything. If we are not learning – then what on earth are we doing?

In retrospect I am aware that in today's culture the behaviour of my parents to make a living, may well be seen as an abuse of my educational needs. At the same time it fed a compulsion to get along quickly and easily with new groups of people combined with an uncanny skill to pick up on learning really quickly. This is how reflection works.

Aside from this there were some other aspects that have driven me forward in a passion for the equality and fairness that appear to have eluded me in some aspects of my life – that is a propulsion to ensure equality for others – particularly for looked after children. I think that many adults of my generation (b. 1957) may have found a lack of attention to the emotional side of their lives or attention to or acknowledgement of an inner life of thoughts and feelings.

It was part of the context in which we lived. Schooling was about basics – not necessarily creatively or emotionally driven. I continue to believe that parents of that era had survived the war and many hardships and prioritised the idea that they were lucky to survive in decent homes with growing amounts of comfort and economic security after living through a period of uncertainty and fear. That was certainly the view in my home – food on the table, order, clean sheets – and the opportunity to play – really this was heaven compared to the bombed east end of London in which my mother was raised in a family of six and my father raised the last child in a family of nine. Since a lack of danger from an external enemy was my mother's focus – why would the emotional lives of her children have much importance, especially when her own had to be systematically ignored!

My mother's childhood was stunted and blighted by the trauma of evacuation and separation in middle childhood and the loss of innocence through constant fear of an invisible enemy raining down on the East End of London – the blitz. Yet in many ways, our emotional lives are the most important functions and manifestation of ourselves. They are the core of our being and a fundamental part of our sensitivity, intelligence and communication. We ignore children's emotions at much cost to them, their mental health and society. How would the former generation have known that, given the minimalist, survival-based conditions of their own lives? My parents certainly did not know this, but they did their very best. As a child under the age of eight, I recall dreaming about the blitz and waking up terrified. I dreamed one night that I had to shelter in a cage under a table. It was not until I was an adult that I realised that I dreamed about my mother's childhood fears of being bombed and having to shelter under the table in a cage. Her distress and trauma had passed unconsciously and without words to the next generation. She would never have been able to talk with me about this and may well have been cross if I had raised the issue of her worst nightmare. For her it was over. For her body and mind – it was far from over.

Of less importance but of great value and significant influence was the slightly adventurous and unbridled nature of myself and my sister – very close in age and often 'let out' to play and explore with none of the constrictions that were present at home relating to orderliness and control. We were subject to a kind of tolerable neglect that probably gave my mother room to breathe and space to think. Nobody knew what we were up to most of the time. I have many memories of joyful play and adventure and yet on reflection we may have been considered quite wild kids who got into problematic situations who should have been subject to more observation and thought and parental control and perhaps attention to the detail of our lives. We were so wild in our explorations that I am very surprised we did not get killed in the process. This is not an exaggeration or romanticism – I still have flashbacks to a frozen pond in the middle of the Cambridgeshire fenlands into which my sister and I both fell when our imaginary ice skates and dramatic dancing led to a sharp cracking of the ice. How we are not still frozen there in time and undiscovered escapes me. The ice kept breaking and cracking under us as we struggled to the side of that pond. We arrived home having run a mile in frozen clothes and were scolded for getting muddy and with no apparent interest for our shock and trauma!

I also freeze a little at the nest of baby snakes that I found when we were exploring in Africa. This is not a metaphor – this was for real and in fact – a nest of cobras. I continue to believe that the female cobra was out for a coffee morning the day that we explored her nest in which her infant cobras were left squirming and writhing around – there must have been six or eight of them. I spent many fascinating moments with a stick and her baby cobras noticing how they reared just like a real spitting cobra with little mini hoods (how cute I thought) but they were only four inches long. Something made me stop suddenly before retreating with some sense that danger was coming. Since I was standing in a monsoon ditch, I would not have been found for some time if I had been bitten and somebody had finally noticed I was missing. In addition to that there was the deadly boomslang snake that slid across my foot in the garden as I went to retrieve our puppy. I think the snake might have been heading for the puppy as a target. Time slowed for a few seconds as I was in such danger, the like of which I would probably never see again. Heaven apparently held me in her arms for a few split seconds. I was totally unaware of the danger until afterwards. Aside from this we were constantly racing down hills on bikes with no brakes or falling off very high haystacks near to farming machinery. None of this killed me, but there were no adult witnesses to the risks which we faced without a second thought.

I wonder if these unfettered moments of childhood, unobserved by adults, made me very concerned for the observation and safety of children; I know only too well just how far children can go with no containment. On the other hand I have pondered that perhaps these moments enhanced my learning and development and helped me to become a creative individual who is happy to think out of the box. And yet in relation to the children we care for with very troubled thoughts and behaviours and abusive experiences of parental harm and intrusion, the experiences of my own childhood would be thought of as very minor incidents. I am aware of the kind of danger from predators and deliberate harm that the children today have been subjected to. The environment seems to be polluted with opportunities for inappropriate sex, violence and mindless behaviour through drugs. It makes falling off a haystack and lack of parental supervision look tame by comparison. The metaphor of the nest of vipers comes rather to have a different meaning. The fundamental difference is that ultimately all of the experiences that I describe from my background gave me spirit and enhanced my sense of survival and love for life and possibly made me quite robust – they did not break my spirit or leave me blunted. In all of these events, however, there is a notable absence of parental interaction and sometimes a lack of awareness and concern. There seemed to be an overriding value, 'Children can take care of themselves.' Actually they cannot and it would be most unfortunate if I brought this value to my work.

This story is not included to tell you all about me, but to give you an example of an act of reflection about how I come to be me.

REFLECTION LEADS TO UNDERSTANDING

It is important that we paint ourselves into the picture when it comes to caring for others. It is not all about us, but on the other hand – something may motivate us to do this work and it is important that we acknowledge that and understand the roots of it so that we have boundaries around ourselves and know exactly where our personal experiences may be influencing us.

Most importantly, we can acknowledge the minds and unique experiences of others – just as we can acknowledge our own. This came to the surface for me very obviously in my doctoral research in which I tried to capture my own life story which emerged as the project progressed. I did this through keeping a reflective diary.

That diary was a reflection on my own attachment experience both then in my childhood and now as an adult – relating to my attachment relationships as they are. I did this because I was aware that my own innate experience of attachment would influence any situation in which I was placed – whether I was a therapist, an educator or simply an observer.

Our attachment experience is always there – always part of the fabric of what we do, coursing through our veins and energetically connecting our body to our brain through electrical impulses and information processing whether it is thought or memory or feeling. Keeping a diary helped me to keep track of this. It was part of a qualitative framework of research in which I learned not to cut out the researcher or pretend there were no researcher effects. Instead, I painted the researcher (myself) into the picture and got clear about what was influencing me. The question was: How did my mental and emotional life impact on the children with whom I was working? That is the question of this book and it is the question of work with children.

That diary, over a year in time, told me many things about myself that I did not even know or understand. It certainly made me realise the potency of our life experience in informing and provoking our thoughts and behaviours. In so many ways we are captive to the circumstances into which we are born – both through our genetic and physical inheritance, our class and even our geography. For example, I had always known that equality was an important aspect of our social world and society, but I had never really understood the importance of that concept or how it impacted on me until I noticed the inequalities in my own upbringing with regard to class and education. As a result of diary keeping I was finally able to acknowledge and recognise in myself the working class experience that I had never thought before had made any difference to my life. But it had.

Being working class brought with it so many disadvantages and yet – in some ways so much insight and understanding and even freedoms and advantages of its own. I was able to acknowledge the painful and uncomfortable reality that life is not an equal playing field. Men and women are not born equal to each other and the class divide means that people have very different experiences of life. Different races have been rendered unequal for many thousands of years as our civilisation develops and whilst we are on the journey to equality – there is still much residual prejudice towards racial difference. We can celebrate a black American president, but this does not wipe away the price that we are paying for the prejudice that has become encoded into our systems both biological, personal, political, educational and social. It is actually very frightening to think just how arbitrary life is and how so much of what we experience is just an accident of birth. My world stopped for a while when I realised that there is nothing fair about the world we live in at all and that there was nothing particularly fair in my own world. Not in terms of my gender, the decade into which I was born, the point in global history to which my parents were subjected or the negligence of adults with regard to my education or emotional life or the type of education that I received.

This chapter is written to demonstrate the process of reflective thought that can lead us from understanding ourselves to understanding others.

Without having given the matter careful thought, I may well have duplicated the values of my upbringing 'Children can take care of themselves' in the work that I do. This idea within my home environment very probably meant that at times I did not receive the attention that I needed or at least the right kind of attention at the right time. Attention is a key nutrient in the life of a child. In fact I am acutely aware that children cannot take care of themselves and need much attention, and the research that I have carried out has helped me to understand this (North 2010).

Being in touch with my story has helped me to understand this deficit to quite an uncomfortable degree.

To conclude, I'd like to reiterate that being in touch with your own biography is neither indulgent nor narcissistic (although it can become this too). It is simply important to be able to observe your own inherited value system to see what you might transfer to others.

If the idea that 'Children can take care of themselves' had been a blind spot for me, I may have become negligent in giving attention to children in my work or my parenting. Instead it has become a helpful and guiding principle – they need support and attention from mindful adults.

SUMMARY

- Our personal experience of attachment is stored in our memory and retrieved at an automatic level. It shows in our behaviours and attitudes and the way that we relate to people. Understanding our life story is a step towards self-reflection and our own personal psychology.

- To pay attention to our own history is part of being mindful. The brain stores historical information

– our history is part of who we were and who we have become. We cannot have a mind that does not have a history (even in cases of bad loss of memory – other people store our history for us).

- We need to be aware of the style of relationship we had in childhood. There will likely be productive and unproductive things that we have learned.

- We can change our values through reflective practice.

- We cannot really accept ourselves if we do not accept our own life story.

- If we show that we are accepting, mindful and correcting of our own lives – we will demonstrate this to the children for whom we care.

- Part of understanding children with complex history is to understand that story for them.

- Children will not necessarily want to access their own history – it is not our job to force children to accept their life story and we may traumatise them if we do this, but this does not mean that we cannot be mindful of the fact that everyone has a history.

- During your own reflective time you could focus on the values and beliefs that you have internalised from childhood – especially those relating to childcare.

- You could note your own style of relating to others now – what is the quality of that style – is it anxious, relaxed, dismissing, joyful or controlling?

Chapter **6**

THE REFLECTIVE PRACTICE PENTAGON

This model sets out a map for supporting reflective practice, and is designed to be a practical tool to aid reflection and help guide your responses and decision-making.

If you sit down to think about an answer to a question you will notice that you tend to only think within very confined limits – tight circles going round and round the central idea until you come out with your preferred solution.

We do not necessarily easily evaluate critically the culture in which we live.

You may think your environment is perfect or feel too threatened by change to notice the things that need to be different. People will often head straight for their mental comfort zone – exactly the opposite response to what reflection and reflexivity is all about.

It is quite natural to want to stay in your comfort zone, but we are all charged with the challenge to develop the critical side of our thinking which enables and motivates us to improve: to make changes that benefit working practices as a whole for the young people for whom we care.

Take the time to learn the skills that enable you to be self-critical or evaluate objectively. Reflective time (sometimes referred to as supervision) can become and is often used as a way to 'tick boxes' and confirm behaviours rather than analyse them, but good supervision is invaluable.

It is extremely helpful to get someone from the outside to think with you and ask the difficult 'what if...' questions; indeed, I'd encourage considering appointing a constructive critic who would be well-placed to encourage you, your team or your organisation to reflect on practice.

The Reflective Practice Pentagon is designed as a prompt or agenda for critical evaluation – helping you to think more broadly and effectively.

There are some very effective models of supervision available which I have found useful, all of which facilitate a 'perspective' on therapeutic work. Peter Hawkins and Robin Shohet wrote the first edition of the classic (and in my opinion unbeatable) *Supervision in the Helping Professions* in 1989 which provides a great map of therapeutic work to include what they call the 'process' model of supervision – it's a model that has endured (Hawkins and Shohet 1989).

Elizabeth Holloway wrote a 'systems' approach to supervision in which she emphasises the ability to think reflexively about the various levels of impact on thinking (Holloway 1995). The Reflective Practice Pentagon I describe below is different in that it has been developed specifically for child-focused work and incorporates a focus on specific areas pertinent to work with children, and in particular for carers to notice what is going on within themselves, especially in relation to emotion regulation and emotional literacy.

The Pentagon also takes into consideration the idea that there are many kinds of person and professional helping in the task of caring for children rather than just counsellors or psychotherapists who traditionally are more individually focused in their work. It draws on the 'building blocks' covered earlier in this book of mindfulness and emotion regulation and is designed to encourage you to notice your own mind and to be 'mind minded'. It provides a simple focus that should help to clarify some of your thinking.

Ultimately I hope that you will travel so much further in your work than just the Pentagon – but it's a starting point.

The Reflective Practice Pentagon

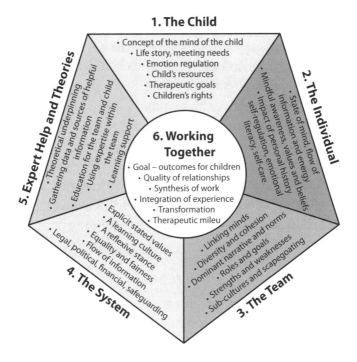

1. SIDE ONE OF PENTAGON: THE CHILD

Putting the child first

Let's put the child first. The Victoria Climbié enquiry in the United Kingdom was the case of a young child whose care was divided between two continents – Africa and Europe. She had been sent to live with her Aunt by her parents in Africa who thought that she would receive the best education and therefore the best start in life. In fact her Aunt treated her cruelly and the child died from maltreatment in 2003.

The Government's initiative *Every Child Matters* was set up following an inquiry into the case which found that the police, the social services departments of four local authorities, the National Health Service and local churches all had contact with her. It was apparent following the judgement in the Victoria Climbié enquiry that a range of professionals failed to understand the circumstances of the care properly. An element of *Every Child Matters* guides childcare practitioners to keep the safety and well-being of children at the front of their mind. In this particular case, nobody noticed what was going on and she was lost in the depths of the social care system.

As professionals working with children, we might feel ashamed or helpless when we think of Victoria's death, but reflecting on the learning has greater potential to help other children.

Thinking holistically about the mind of the child

- How do you think about this child or young person in your care?

- How are you understanding their behaviour?

- Are you really understanding their motivation or are you perhaps just making assumptions based on their behaviour?

- Ask yourself, how are you holding the child in your mind? Draw on your understanding of mindfulness to be 'mind minded': what is in your mind when you are thinking about this child?

A holistic conceptualisation involves many elements which are described below under the heading, 'holding the child in mind'.

Here are some questions you could ask under the heading of 'mind-minded' care:

Holding the child in mind

- What do you think this child or young person/patient is thinking about their life?

- Does this child have a specific mental health problem?

- Is this child anxious?

- Is this child traumatised?

- How is that trauma being acted out or affecting this child or those around this child?

- How does this child form relationships – are they afraid to trust others?

- Are they manipulative?

- Can you identify clearly the qualities of this child's relational style?

- Is this young person afraid to rely on adults for care?

- Does this young person have a learning difficulty or disability that we need to consider?

- Does this young person express emotion or do they act out their inner life through behaviour?

- What information do we have about this young person's attempts to communicate? What is the result?

- Does this young person need to develop emotional literacy? How can we help him/her?

- What activities does this young person like?

- What events brought this young person into your care?

- What is this young person good at and what do they like doing?

- What or who is this young person most afraid of?

- Who does this young person hate the most or feel most angry towards?

- Has this child been running away? What do we think they are running from?

How to use these questions

Sit down and write your reflections on these questions. Reflect on them yourself, or share them with colleagues. The process or sharing can help you to develop a sense of how accurate your assumptions are and enable you to formulate a clear conceptualisation of both the child's behaviour and inner life.

Finally try asking yourself the following question: 'How is this child's inner life of thoughts and feelings linked to their behaviour?'

This is just the start of your understanding and it could take weeks or even months to establish the full picture. You could then move on to other areas of focus and information gathering.

History of the child's life

You cannot understand a child or young person in your care if you do not have a chronology or historical account of their life.

If you do not have an accurate life story or history then you can only make assumptions about the child's experiences, and they may well be wrong. As a carer it is essential that you show a young person that you are interested in their story – it is one of the main features of therapeutic/supportive care.

You will note that I place great emphasis on stories and life narratives in this book – our own and those of our children. If we know and accept our life story with all of its highs and lows (sometimes extreme) then we will be more likely to accept ourselves and be managing, correcting, adjusting and regulating our lives.

A child may not wish to recall or remember their own story. It may have been so difficult or painful that they prefer to forget. This has to be respected. However you may still need to know that story in order to help that child. You don't have to keep reminding them of the things they don't want to remember. But you do have to hold that story in your mind for the child as it will tell you about him or her. Whether you have an accurate chronology or not it is always best to gain the child's view of their life so far and this can be achieved through a simple time line drawing. This may take some time to achieve and could trigger lots of thought and conversation with the child.

Life story gathering needs to be a focused and specialised time – not just a snatched conversation. We need to demonstrate that we give priority to this information. Here are some guidelines for thinking about the standards to achieve in terms of the type of information you will need to gather in a history.

Information gathering about the child's history

- A history should describe the child's parents, and their state of mind, behaviours and experiences of their relationship around the conception and birth of the child. It should describe in detail all the home circumstances of that child. If the history is given by the child themselves it will of course describe their view of this.

- It should describe the social conditions of the child's birth and the health conditions at birth – also any health conditions of the birth parents, i.e. drug and alcohol abuse, poverty, mental health problems, domestic violence, criminality, corruption etc. These things will have had impact on the child in your care.

- It should tell you about both chronological events and also emotional and attachment events. Chronological events are historical, linear and factual such as house moves and changes in schools (remember left brain?). Emotional events are relational changes (remember right brain?) such as separations from family and births of family members or other losses such as deaths in the family. It should describe attachment events such as the parents changing partners, loss of parents or loss of family members such as siblings as well as pets.

- The chronology should describe traumatic events that have caused harm, abuse or upset to the child. For example if a child has been physically abused, abandoned or rejected – these things do have an impact and must be considered especially in relation to the child's behaviour.

- The chronology should give details of subsequent carers from social care such as foster carers or kinship carers. There should be details of the quality of these relationships. You should know if the child was abused whilst in Local Authority care – this may make a huge impact on the care that you subsequently give to the child (and whether or not the child will want to trust adults). You should also know when they have had wonderful and really supportive substitute carers – as this will also make an impact and children can safely link back to memories of those people.

- If children have been running away you should be able to provide an explanation of possible events that might lead to that. After an event of running away there should be an interview with the child to help with understanding. Running away means something in the child's mind.

- You should know the whereabouts of parents who are now separated from the child. You should also be told if those parents are missing or dead or if they have just chosen not to be in touch with the child.

- The rule is that history matters – especially attachment history and the history of care. It will be coursing through the child's life, brain and mind as a flow of information and energy and informing their thinking. It is helpful to the child to support them with their story as it emerges if they demonstrate that they wish to do this.

Developmental stage

As described earlier in this book a common parenting/carer error is to make mistakes about what a child can achieve; a failure to take into consideration the child's actual capacity.

Children may be functioning at a level that is lower than their chronological age. There is no harm in offering developmental age-appropriate support to a child who is functioning at a younger age.

Common mistakes relate to assumptions about a child's ability to care for themselves or to be more independent. Adult frustrations about these behaviours can be distressing to a child, and could be considered as emotionally abusive.

When working with vulnerable children and young people it is better to initially under- than to over-estimate a child's developmental age and capability. A child who has had the right amount of supportive dependence on adults will often achieve just the right amount of autonomy and self-care. A child who is dismissed by adults as being able to care for themselves will often not care properly for themselves in the long term. We all need support at times and there is no harm whatsoever in supporting a child in activities and behaviours that we may think of as 'younger' than their years.

For example, if a 12-year-old is not cleaning their teeth properly, there is nothing to be lost by standing with them when they clean their teeth so that they get it right. Older children need hugs as well as younger children (as long as it is made explicitly clear that it is not a sexualised hug). Older children may need help with organising their clothes and their rooms and it is supportive to do these tasks with them (if you are given permission to go in their room). Here are some helpful guidelines.

Chronological age/developmental age

The following questions are designed to help you reflect on whether or not you are attending to a child's developmental stage appropriately.

- Do I know what is appropriate for a child of this age?

- Does the child have a recognised developmental or learning difficulty?

- Has the child regressed, and are they needing care as if they are a younger child?

- Have I got any framework at all for child development?

- Do teenagers still need nurturing? How would I do this in an age-appropriate way?

- What if an older teenager refuses to work towards independence?

- What sort of attachment experience can these young people expect?

- What do we do with a child who appears to need no care at all?

- What if a child keeps forgetting things – how do I support them?

Current attachment relationships

Here are some questions to help you reflect on the attachment relationship of the child.

Attachment relationships always have an effect on a child – even if it is just for that child to completely deny that it has any affect at all. The child may not want to know about their birth parents and we have to respect this. However, as a carer or supporter you do need to hold these relationships in mind for the future for the child. At times you have to hold things in mind for the child that they cannot hold in mind for themselves or do not wish to think about. This should be seen as part of the supportive role.

- Where are the birth parents? What are they doing and what happened to those parents? What are the realistic chances of rehabilitation?

- Where or when did separation occur and why did it occur? This always has an impact.

- What do you think the effect is with your particular child?

- Did this child feel rejected or are they hurt by rejection?

- Does this child still miss those parents – if you don't know how will you find out?

- What is the child's fantasy about those parents – what are they imagining?

- How can you work with this child or young person to show them that you value their thoughts and feelings about their attachment relationships, whether they are positive or negative?

Obvious needs and less obvious needs

Deprived children and young people may obscure their real needs because they are used to hiding them from adults – emotional, physical and mental; often their needs for safety and love.

For example, a 16-year-old may need a teddy on his bed even though he would never admit it – how would you set about providing for those kinds of needs without causing shame or humiliation?

Reflect on how you think about this sort of emotional need – do you think it is babyish or are you willing to work with it?

You must have a coherent plan in order to meet these needs. What about things like a milky drink at bed-time to provide nurturing, slippers to show that you care how warm or cold a child might be, getting a child to wear a coat in the cold – even though they would prefer to shiver. These details are the most important yet hidden and subtle aspect of therapeutic childcare work. If you spend a lot of time working out such needs on a daily basis you will show to the child that you care.

The general rule is that if you meet a need, it is generally likely to subside and move a child forward (Griffin and Tyrrell 2011). If you ignore a need, it is likely to contribute towards that child or young person remaining needy and stuck in that need. People can be arrested in their needs for their whole lives. Meeting needs will release the potential for a child to receive care.

Human needs revolve around the following, so try to think in all of these areas. Maslow's hierarchy of needs is a useful framework for understanding human needs and behaviours (Maslow 1943), but Griffin and Tyrrell's *Human Givens* is also a solid and more modern model of human needs (Griffin and Tyrrell 2011).

1. Safety and survival.

2. Nurturing.

3. Support.

4. Food and water.

5. Love and affection.

6. Achievement.

7. Actualisation.

It is also helpful to understand our emotional needs. The list of emotional needs below are also from *Human Givens* (Griffin and Tyrrell 2011, p.93).

- Security.

- Attention.

- Autonomy and self-management.

- Emotionally connected to others.

- Being part of a wider community.

- The need for friendship and intimacy.

- A sense of status.

- A sense of competence.

- A sense of meaning and purpose.

Current challenges in behaviour and consequences table

Consider the following:

- How are you responding to challenging behaviour?

- Is it making you cross?

- Does it leave you defeated?

In order to help a child who is troubled you need to show them that you can manage and meet the challenge, you need to be secure and show good self-management, show that you know right from wrong, and provide a consequence if necessary.

You need to avoid being weak on one hand, and over-controlling on the other. If you respond weakly a child will take advantage, be out of control and will probably not feel safe. If you respond with too much control, a child will become angry and aggressive. The key word is *authority*. Even if you don't feel it you need to respond with a confident authoritative manner at all times. If you don't feel confident, then take advice and get support.

Dan Hughes has an excellent formula for the stance of a carer – he refers to PLACE: Playful, loving, accepting, curious and empathic (Hughes 1998). It is helpful to remember PLACE, as a formula for reminding you how to respond at difficult times.

In the course of undertaking a research project, I consulted with one of my carers, who came up with a formula that she referred to as 'kind, calm and caring'. She noticed that if she adopted this stance even at times of extreme difficulty she was likely to have a better outcome (North 2010).

An authoritative, calm response will help in all situations, and reflective practice should play a key part in nurturing calm and authority. Reflecting on the following questions will help ongoing evaluation and self-management in order to support the child.

- What are the current challenges being shown by this child or young person?

- What is this young person trying to communicate by this behaviour?

- What are the consequences for this behaviour?

- Are the consequences meaningful and effective, helping the young person to learn, or are they punishing?

- How are you in your authoritative stance?

The child's fears and vulnerabilities

We all have fears and vulnerabilities. Invincible and tough children will sometimes be able to convince us that they do not. They are often the most frightened children. All children have the right to be protected and often the most invulnerable, tough and aggressive children are the children who have not been protected. So don't be fooled that some children appear to be unafraid – it is never ever true.

Often a child's greatest fear is that they will be humiliated or put to shame and they will fight off a sense of shame. A physical fight or facing outward danger might be preferable to the awful feelings of aloneness and despair that arise out of shame. Our actions should not therefore be shaming, but should be educational for children. That is why we need to think so carefully around the children for whom we care. Here are some questions to assist the process of thinking about fear.

- What are your own worst fears and how might you defend yourself from feeling shame and vulnerability?

- What fears do you think this child has?

- Is there a way you can help them feel less afraid and more secure?

- How do a child's fears affect their behaviour?

The child's emotional states

As with fear, we all have emotional states. Our emotions are an expression of our responses to life – fear, love, anger, happiness, disgust, shame, jealousy, surprise and interest. Learning attachment theory shows us that it is through helping children with their emotions that we help them to have a happy mental life and to feel secure. It is through helping children deal with emotional states that we help them to mature emotionally and not remain ensnared in painful cycles of thought and behaviour.

We also need to help our children in care towards more authentic happiness based on a sense of belonging and security – not based on the latest computer game or designer label acquisition. True happiness in a child will increase confidence and self-esteem and help a child feel that they have the resources to cope. This is our most important task.

Ask yourself:

- What is the predominant emotional state in this child?

- How can you help this child to feel happier and more confident?

- How does this child manage emotion? Suppression of emotion is not management.

- Who in particular does this child turn to with emotional states – what can you learn from that person? How do you prevent that person from becoming isolated?

- Are you helping this child with emotional literacy – helping them to talk about their emotional states and name their emotions?

- Are you emotionally literate yourself – locating a sense of what you feel at any given moment in time – informing your actions? Do you actually value emotions as our friends or do you drive them away as a nuisance?

- What can you learn from this child's predominant states?

The child's skills and positive resources, achievements and resilience

Sometimes when children are having a difficult time we can get lost in the negatives because of the impact on us. It is helpful to have a clear list of the child's achievements and abilities and all the good things that have happened in their lives as well as the best aspects of their behaviour. It may be good to help a child to compile this list with you and keep it in a place where they can see it often. It is easy to get stuck in the negatives of life and many children with negative experiences need our help and support with a way out from these. We need to help children and young people to visualise or consider the positives – at least daily. Here is some guidance to supporting positive states.

- Make a house rule that everyone (including you) has to come up with three positives in their day. Whilst at the same time being able to...

  - acknowledge any real difficulties that a child is experiencing...whilst at the same time

  - help a child to see any negatives from a new perspective for example 'areas for learning'.

- Have a list of your own general positives including your behaviour.

- Help the child have a list of positives on their wall in their room or in a place of their choosing. (They may or may not want to share this.)

- Engage in activities at which the child can win. This reinforces positive states.

- Help to frame events in a positive way rather than a negative way.

- Help a child to see others in a positive way rather than a negative way.

- Comfort a child if they feel anxious or upset – before you help them move on to the positives.

However, these suggestions do not apply to any tragedy or real upset in the child's life such as death of a pet, a loved one or loss of someone special. These are times when a lot of support is needed.

Goals for the future and a therapeutic plan

Consult with other professionals on the proposed therapeutic plan for the child.

If you are making your own plan then ensure clear, realistic short-term goals that are achievable and not setting the child up to fail (often referred to as SMART goals – Specific, Measurable, Achievable, Realistic and set within a Time frame).

Don't be afraid to set the bar lower rather than higher as this will strengthen motivation and encourage enthusiasm. Help the child to be mindful of their own plan and most of all help the child to come up with their own realistic and achievable goals. Change may be behavioural, emotional (anger management) or mental (changing attitudes). If you are stuck for goals, then some general guidelines are:

- Working towards happier states of mind through positive experiences.

- Suggesting daily healthy activities in which the child can be involved.

- Supporting the child to manage behaviour appropriately.

- Helping the child to become more reflective about events.

- Improving management of emotional states.

- Working on emotional literacy (ability to name and label thoughts and feelings).

- Supporting the child with their life and helping them to allow support.

- Evaluating the developmental stage of the child and helping them to meet developmental goals.

2. SIDE TWO OF PENTAGON: THE INDIVIDUAL

The key words for this side of the Pentagon are awareness and state of mind. In order to manage successfully the task of managing children with complex needs, we have to be acutely self-aware – this means awareness of our own thoughts, feelings and reactions.

The task of caring for children requires that adults do not overlook the importance of human interaction, and not to pretend that they are working in a factory and that the work of caring is mechanical. Children who need therapeutic care are complex, because their needs have not been met and they have often been harmed by adults. Therefore carers have to present themselves to children as uniquely human, but also have to show that they are self-managing, reflective agents who are *safe* people.

In the process of interacting with children, sensitivity to them matters more than anything else. Here is an example of how reflective practice may help in a difficult scenario. If a child you are caring for is in a bad temper and kicks you, your natural reaction might be to become defensive or worse still kick back, get cross or call the police. However, those working therapeutically with children are required to think before acting: to control your response, self-soothe and at the same time attempt to understand the mind of the child who has just given you a good kick.

This is a lot to ask of any human being as it is going against your natural and instinctive reactions to protect yourself. The stance that needs to be adopted in this kind of scenario is that of an authoritative, compassionate, reflective individual. That is not to say you cannot verbalise the process to a child. You might say, 'You have really hurt me and I am going to take time to deal with my leg. When I feel better I would like to talk to you about this.' You may of course have strong feelings about being kicked. You would be expected to deal with those feelings in the reflective arena with a supervisor – and we would expect such a supervisor or manager to be very compassionate and supportive towards you. The rule is that you cannot give what you do not get, and you cannot teach if you do not know.

We therefore also have to be supportive of each other through such times as being kicked so that we do not harden our hearts to the children we work with. It is not good practice to 'forget about it', nor is it safe to become immune to being kicked. The way to go is to reflect on the experience and put it in its place.

I can recall being told by one member of a team that 'she would deal with things in her own way'. This team member had a strong aversion to any kind of reflective practice. I knew this would be a problem and however I tried to persuade her of the value of thinking things through, she would not engage. I was not surprised when months later I heard that the same person had lashed out at a child and was of course removed from their post. It was a very sad outcome for everyone concerned, primarily for the child who had just found someone else they could not trust to keep them safe.

Another team member caring for a troubled child was actually bitten badly on the arm when on duty. She went to hospital and her wounds were dealt with. Fortunately there was no infection and the bite was not too deep. Without being asked she was in my office the next morning to talk her experience through. It had deeply troubled and upset her. We spent some days helping her with her state of mind and her reactions to this. The team member returned to work with the clear intention of showing the child concerned that she had survived the assault. The child was devastated that he had hurt her and collapsed into her arms. Rather than dismiss him out of revenge she was fully ready to help him learn from the harm he had caused. She was not pleased, but she understood that the child had to learn quickly from this serious assault. That member of the team was able to cope with the child's feelings and help him to learn from his aggressive reaction. Her response was exceptional. Had she not felt able to let go and move on from any thoughts of revenge, an alternative solution would have been to allow that carer to go to another unit for work until she had found her resources again. As it was, time spent in reflective practice promoted her already exceptional resources and she showed the child a remarkable response. I have no doubt that the experience will stay with that child for the rest of his life and will have had more impact on his mind than any rough justice which may have proved another opportunity for rejection.

What is it then that you are expected to be reflective about? Here are some outlines for your guidance. We hope that you will add your own areas for further thought as you discover them.

Your own values and beliefs

Your mind and personality could be described as the sum total of your values and core beliefs about the world. Here are some questions to help you to reflect on your values and beliefs.

- What are the three things that most matter to you in your life?

- What are your goals for your life?

- Ultimately what are the three most important things that you believe about people and the world you live in?

- Name three people whom you respect the most – what is it that you respect about those people? What qualities do you admire?

- Think of someone you find it hard to respect. State clearly what it is your find hard to respect about that person.

- If you died – how would you like people to remember you and what would you think you had contributed to your life? What three things do you think you would be remembered for?

Our experiences at work

Reflecting on your experiences at work and the predominant states of mind that your job involves will help you to have a more considered and well-managed response.

You will have your public thoughts at work and you will have your private thoughts about your job. Of course your private thoughts are your own, but be aware for yourself how your private values may affect your outcomes at work. For example, do you think you will 'manage things your own way?' If this is the case – what is 'your own way?'

Consider:

- What does this job mean to you?

- How do work experiences affect you? Do they make you feel down, frustrated? What is your predominant emotion about your work?

- What do you really think about the child or young person you work with?

- What further information do you need to help you to understand this child?

- What do you really think about your team members?

- How can you frame your difficulties constructively with team members?

- Think of the person you get on with the least. How could you improve this relationship?

- What are the highs and lows of your day?

- Is it more low than high?

- Do you just forget about experiences of work when you get home?

- Or do you spend hours thinking about what has happened?

There is a second level to the idea of experience – that is the experience from your own life that has given you information about how to cope. This could be called your internal working model on life (Bowlby 1988).

We all bring with us a set of experiences relating to being cared for by others in childhood. These may be positive or negative and will very probably be a mixture of both as no parent is perfect all the time. This is an inevitable part of being human and that is why we ask our practitioners to be in touch with their own story because life experiences inform our values and belief systems.

Take an example: what might a person do if they were brought up to think that slapping helps children to behave? This is not a helpful idea, particularly when working with vulnerable children, but remains a commonly held belief. However, through reflexive and reflective practice you can become aware of it and manage and correct this incorrect belief. To move from the idea of slapping a child for being naughty to helping a child reflect on what had gone wrong, you would need to have more knowledge and information.

Here are some questions to help you to think about that:

- What were the three main things that you learned about behaviour in your childhood?

- What are the three most negative beliefs that you may transfer from your childhood learning?

- What are the three most positive beliefs that you may transfer from your childhood learning?

- What experience from childhood has a positive impact on your work?

- What experience from childhood has a negative impact on your work?

- Name the three best qualities of the person on whom you could rely the most.

- Name the three most negative qualities of the person on whom you could rely the least.

Our thoughts feelings

Thoughts are going through our mind all of the time – often they are submerged just below our consciousness.

What do we think about events? What do we think of how our colleagues are managing things? What is the best way to manage a difficult situation? How could we manage it better next time? What are we planning for tea tonight? What is worrying us about the next few hours?

Ultimately our thoughts and feelings will be visible in our behaviour. Earlier in the book, I have described mindfulness, and the mind as being a piece of predictive machinery which is constantly trying to control and make sense of every moment of our lives. It constantly asks, 'What is the best next move for my optimum survival right now?' Be more aware of the thoughts and feelings that are flowing through your mind at any given moment in time. It takes a small amount of time (perhaps 20 minutes) to sit and collect your thoughts about how you are right now.

Concerns raised as questions

Ideally we should all work in an environment in which we could freely voice any concerns about the work we are involved in and have them considered. If you do not work in this kind of enlivening environment, you might want to ask why. If you cannot voice your concerns to your team, you should at least be able to voice them privately to your manager or another senior member of staff within your organisation and they should welcome your thoughts on your work. These concerns may range from the subtle and small, and certainly should always relate to safety and protection of children and the way that we go about our job, or they may be major concerns. The first step to resolving problems should be to ask questions and raise the issue of concern. You may not of course get the exact solution that you desire, but raising questions about problems is a fundamental right and the basis of a healthy organisation that is full of curiosity and enquiry.

Our belonging in the team

Each team needs to learn to value its individual members and their own unique contribution. Any team that is scapegoating (blaming one individual) is neither processing information or responding reflectively, and certainly not learning. The opposite of scapegoating is reflecting and understanding the problems. Here are some areas that you could start to consider.

- How can you ask your team to support you?

- Do you value all members of the team?

- How can you support them better?

- Do you think your team fully understand your strengths and vulnerabilities?

- Do you take responsibility for getting your needs met – or do you moan and complain?

Our emotional states at work and at home

Yes, your emotional states at work do matter. You are not going to feel like the sun is shinning every day. But you could consider the following:

- How do the emotional states of the child I care for affect me?

- Am I acting pro-actively to manage my own emotions?

- Do I have a predominant emotion that I bring to work?

- Am I contributing to a happier workplace environment?

- Do I believe that this matters anyway?

- Where can I find out more information about creating positive states?

- How do I help the child I care for with authentic emotional states?

- Is there something personal that has affected me that I may bring to work that is not helpful? How do I manage this?

Individual learning and self-care plan

Everyone in the team should have an individual learning and self-care plan set out clearly with goals. Do not expect to be involved in social pedagogy or therapeutic childcare without a learning and development plan for yourself. You could ask yourself a question – if you are not learning – then what are you doing? The agenda should be set by you and it can relate to whatever you want in your personal development as well as development in the job. They may tie in together or they may be separate. Central to this learning is the notion of self-care for carers; we cannot care for others unless we are in good condition ourselves. We need to model self-respect, self-regulation and self-acceptance to the young people we care for. This self-care will reveal itself to others in a range of behaviours from the way that we present ourselves to others – for example, in the clothes that we wear. I don't mean that we have to wear designer clothes to be worthy of respect, but we can come to work in clean fresh clothing that shows that we know that these things matter. But our self-respect is also demonstrated in the way that we manage ourselves, and the way that we deal with problems, and the way that we speak about things. As we have learned already in this book, children will pick up on our state of mind very quickly.

Here are a few ideas for you on a personal level or self-care of learning:

- stress management

- self-presentation

- anger management

- money management

- emotional management

- increasing happiness

- emotional literacy

- listening skills

- reflective skills

- health issues: smoking less, drinking less, getting more exercise, eating well.

Here are some ideas for your development on a professional level:

- NVQs

- relevant theories

- social skills training for children

- child development training

- communication skills
- life skills training
- mindfulness training
- Open University courses
- self-development courses.

3. SIDE THREE OF PENTAGON: THE TEAM

A team working together is a complex machine that needs as much attention as the individuals who contribute to that team. Any group of people can be greater than the sum of their parts if they work skilfully together. The key issue is – what is it like for a child to be cared for by our team? What if that group of people had different levels of understanding and skill? It would be even more unsettling for the child we were caring for if people were not thinking in a coherent and uniform way. We cannot hope to be all the same, and we will all bring diversity to the team – however, there must be some cohesion, predictability and uniformity in what we present on a daily basis. In addition, any child who is anxious about hostility and potential conflict as most children in care might be, will pick up immediately as soon as there is any conflict within the team. Troubled and anxious children are quick to spot any cracks that begin to open in their care, especially if they are filled with negativity. For these reasons we have to be pro-active, conscious and constantly on the lookout for areas where we might fail. It is not just the job of the manager or team leader to be looking at the state of the team. It is up to each individual to speak their own truth so that any manager can do their job to the best of their ability.

Here are some areas for reflection. If you keep your eye on these areas you are less likely to become unconscious of the dynamics of the team. The rule is – the dynamics and quality of relationships within the team will be parallel to the quality of the care for our young people. Are those dynamics healthy, powerful and supportive and inspiring – or are they stuck, lacking in joy and spontaneity and simply a mirror of dysfunctional human relationships? The team has its own mind that is made up of all the minds that contribute to it – is that a healthy mind flowing with energy and information? Questions to ask:

- What are we like when we function at our best?

- What are we like when we function at our worst?

- Do we work well with authority and respect our manager?

- How can we support one another at stressful times?

- What behaviours of the child impose the most stress on the team (i.e. aggression)?

- Does the team pick up on the child's negative expectations of adults?

- Do we act out in our team or are we aware of what we are doing?

- What would it be like to be cared for by our team?

Diversity and equality monitoring

Expect difference. Enjoy diversity within your team and pay attention to any sense of leaving out or excluding anyone who is in a minority grouping. Obvious areas are race and culture, gender, religion, sexual orientation or ethnicity. If you have racial and cultural diversity within your team then you will be blessed with a richer range of life experience. Equality is the key word to managing the diversity of the team. There should be no special people, no special cases, no one who is above and beyond the rules of the team. All should have a healthy respect and curiosity for exploring how we as humans are all different. On the other hand, we should be able to identify the unique contribution of each individual. All people within the team should have the same rights. A sense of understanding equality and equal rights is essential to living in the twenty-first century – despite the fact that there are still many anomalies in the world that we inhabit. We do not necessarily live in a fair world and there are plenty of examples of remaining prejudice throughout our world.

Lack of attention to equality can undermine people's confidence and well-being. Think about these things and struggle with them during team reflective time. More importantly think about how the young person in your care manages equality, their rights and diversity. How much help and modelling do they need from the team? Watch out for who you are laughing at or making fun of and be careful that a team 'joke' about someone is not experienced as team bullying. Something that is funny once may not be funny if it makes a person feels isolated or alone, such as laughing at someone's accent or personal tendencies. The rule for diversity is, 'Walk a mile in that person's moccasins.' Watch out for your personal prejudices and notice how you pre-judge people for being different from yourself. If you really explore prejudice it is often based on untrue beliefs that are simply unfair.

The dominant narrative

Every team will have its group thinking (or narrative). The dominant narrative means, 'The things that we continually talk and think about and take for granted.' For example, what is the dominant narrative about equality between men and women – are there subtle sexist jokes or sexist behaviours? Who creates the narrative in your group? Is it created by cliques or by being resistant to moving forward? Is it created by you or is it created by difficult behaviour from a child? What is the source of your information? Is it good information, is your thinking based on myth or reality? Is your narrative sexist? Fatist? Racist? Or is your common thinking created in a reflective environment where you think carefully before you act for and on behalf of others.

Roles and goals within the team

Spend time reflecting on the individual contributions that each member of the team can make. This is also attention to diversity. Everyone will play a different role. Is there a role that the children ask you to play – the bad guy? The compassionate one? The clever one? Are there roles that you play naturally – the chef? The economist? The survival expert? The nurse? Whilst we need to value each contribution and we will all have innate tendencies – do we ever want to swop roles so that they are not solely occupied by one person? If we are aware of the role that we play in the team, we will be more aware of the dynamics or flow of energy throughout the team.

Strengths and weaknesses evaluation

Many teams have started off their reflective practice thinking that they are 'just fine, thank you very much' and then been amazed to discover just how much they have to learn. It is perfectly acceptable to be told that a team is 'happy and working well' and always good news. However, there is always something to learn and I think it is important to exercise caution against this possible defence of 'everything is fine'. 'We are all happy' does not mean there is not something to learn. It is all about learning. What may be a problem is where a team thinks they are just fine and that they have nothing to learn. The team then becomes like a child that will not change its behaviour. The rule is this: We all have our strengths and weaknesses and we all have to develop our skills; no one is exempt from this rule. So spend time evaluating your individual strengths and weaknesses by making a list. Ask your team for support with developing your weaknesses. Then as a team make a list of your team strengths and weaknesses. For example, you may wish to work on your communication skills within the team. You may want to consider your 'blind spots'. You can then congratulate yourselves on how well you are doing because you will have developed a learning plan.

Dyads, cliques and sub-cultures and other threats to a healthy team

It is normal, natural and even healthy that you will get on with some members of the team and form close and abiding friendships. There will always be people to whom you are drawn more than others. However, in real team work you will not sacrifice the working of the team for your preferred friendships. You always have to be thinking of the impact of your preferred friends on the working of the team. All you have to do is consider the impact. Of course you will have close friends, but you have to be aware of how you form closed little groups or 'dyads and duos' to the exclusion of all others, because this will have an impact on the team.

Another common error in a team is for little cliques of people to form around areas of discontent and complaint. This is not healthy team dynamics. If you have a complaint – get it out there – into the team and find a way to manage it together. You have a choice – you can spend years moaning about what is not right or you can spend some time working together to put it right. A clique can form a sub-culture which goes against the healthy and powerful dynamic of a fully functioning team. There is nothing wrong with a sub-group with a specialism or particular interest – say for example, an interest such as sport or politics. But within team work there is a need to make that interest part of the team working, at least while you are at work. Watch out for the 'closed culture' which will damage your team. You need all doors and windows to be open to healthy transparent communication. Closed behaviour is a threat to a healthy team and a threat to the quality of care of children you care for.

Scapegoating

Scapegoating is a threat to a healthy team and a sign that something has gone wrong with the team structure. It is the unacceptable face of blame. It means that someone within your team gets the blame for everything that goes wrong. If you are scapegoating anyone within your team then you are getting something seriously wrong and you are not working as an honest and responsible, transparent and reflective team. Scapegoating is a primitive response to complex problems. You could also be open to the charge of bullying, because blaming one person for everything is unrealistic, dishonest and not taking responsibility; it is also abusive and harmful. Scapegoating is unhealthy practice. It is not good modelling in our line of work and is a highly undesirable dynamic. If someone is getting something wrong then within the spirit of a learning organisation they need to be told about it so that they can get it right and be given the chance to put that right. Scapegoating – don't do it. If you are doing it, do something to put it right now: how about insisting that everyone within the team takes responsibility for the thing that is going wrong? Scapegoating behaviour is a threat to the quality and integrity of your team and a poor model of human behaviour for the children you care for.

Team cohesion: responses to critical incidents and opportunities for learning

Your team will become strong and powerful as you learn more together based on a healthy structure developed from accurate information that you construct together. This includes evaluating and reflecting on your responses as a group to any critical incidents – of which there will be many if you are caring for young people who have had difficult lives. These critical incidents are all opportunities for rich learning about yourselves as individuals and within your team. In your team time you need to constantly reflect on these critical incidents in order to learn from them and for the young people. But you need to be able to do this without causing blame or shame to people. Any blame or need to take responsibility for problems needs to be dealt with privately by managers. The issue within a team is: who is responsible for which part of the incident and what have you learned from that? It is not safe to be open and honest about mistakes in a blame and shame culture. On the other hand it is not safe to work in a culture where people do not take responsibility for themselves and for their actions.

Consider the following:

- What was the incident?

- How did it affect people?

- What did it mean to you as an individual – and the team as a whole?

- How can your team support you in this incident?

- Is there any further learning – do you need any advice? Do you need information or expertise?

- What does this tell us about the child we care for?

- What can we help them to learn from this?

- Are there any safeguarding/health and safety issues?

Reflexivity, responses to the outside world, consistency and information sharing

A team is not a unit on its own; it is not a little island in the great sea of life. This is another common error. It can feel so cosy in your team that you can cut yourself off from the bigger picture and your connections with the outside world and operate by your own rules. Whilst it may feel comfortable, it will ultimately lead to a problem because of insularity and lack of awareness and fresh information.

Your system will become stale and eventually dysfunctional if you are not constantly learning from fresh data. Just as children have to learn to deal with the outside world, so teams also have to respond effectively to the demands of the bigger system. What would be the point of being a joyful little team who are not contributing all of their learning to the other teams in any larger group? We have to have an open and transparent sharing with the bigger organisation as this again is what a learning organisation is all about.

At another level, you have to respond to the laws of the land as well as the general rules of the organisation to which the team belongs. If you find yourself at any stage thinking that it is just 'our little team against the world' then you are probably forgetting to relate to the outside world effectively. A healthy rule would be: information is for sharing – what our are sources of information? Also enquiring of each other – what is going on out there? What are the other teams doing? Who just had a brilliant experience that they want to share? One mistake is to think as a team, 'We know what is best for this child.' It may well be that you know the child very well but it is a mistake to think that you cannot take further advice from the outside world into consideration. Here are some outside systems to think about and include into your thinking. Reflexivity is about including into your thinking the impact from the outside world.

- Children's rights.

- Safeguarding and protection.

- Health systems.

- Social services.

- Legal and law, police, courts and youth offending.

- Voluntary services and charities.

- Professional bodies.

4. SIDE FOUR OF PENTAGON: THE SYSTEM

This is sometimes referred to as a systemic approach to understanding and reflecting on your work. Whilst you have extended your knowledge and awareness to the team system, if you are responding reflexively you will take your knowledge and learning further and include the greater system within your reflective process. Ignoring the system in which you exist would be like a pilot getting in an aircraft and forgetting to notice whether or not there were any air traffic controllers out there for him to relate with during his flight. Many people are woefully unaware of the huge interlinking machinery of our world and thereby seriously disadvantaged and disempowered. You can be confident that systems will impact on the children in your care. As adults who care, we are there to protect children from negative influences such as poverty, war or famine. We are also there to help them relate to and understand how the world works.

We are part of many systems. We are part of a planetary system, a weather system and ecosystem, a financial and economic system, a religious system, an educational system – all such systems have control and influence over us without us even noticing. Mostly these systems consist of constrains on our behaviours and they certainly impact on our thoughts and feelings. To a large extent these systems are immovable and quite lawful – what about the planetary system and the way that it impacts on planet earth. The moon influences the way that the tides change – there is nothing we can do about changing these systems, but we can at least register the impact that they have on us. In most countries one may see how religion influences the development of the legal system, how economics affects the price of food and how politics affects people's ability to earn and support their family.

You could think of family systems as a way of understanding the family that you came from, or the family that the child in your care has emerged from. You could also think of the organisational system in which you exist. It is too easy to complain about organisational systems without making an effort to understand the system and even befriend and work with that system, learning how it has developed and on what philosophical basis it has been built. This can easily be done by looking at the Mission Statement for the organisation. You may find yourself constantly complaining about your organisation, thus wasting a lot of energy with no positive outcome. Do you need to ask some questions about that system so that you can work within it with more acceptance? If a child in your care notices that you are railing against the system, what might you be teaching them about how to cope with the social world? Would it be better to model a willingness to communicate and understand and work with and negotiate the systems with which we have to live? Thinking about and understanding the systems in which you exist is a way to empower yourself and increase your knowledge and understanding of your world. It will also help to empower the child you care for.

One significant area is that of 'rights' for the citizen and in our job this particularly refers to the rights of children. I have found this to be so important in my work that I have included an Appendix to this book in which I reproduce the United Nations (Unicef) Convention on the Rights of Children. We have observed that children who are cared for by the state do not live on the even playing field that a child might experience if they are cared for by loving parents. Sometimes it is hard to bring the rights of children to everyone's attention, but it is important that we do so. Children who are significantly disempowered in their lives in terms of not having a parent onside with them need our help and support, and it is best that we are well equipped with as much knowledge as possible about their needs. So we advise that if you do nothing else with regard to reflexivity in your work that as a minimum you pay attention to the rights of children. If you want to do far more than the bare minimum, we have a list of areas below on which you could reflect as a team.

Ultimately systems are in place to safeguard and support living and standards of care. They uphold ethics in our work together. Ethics is a complicated area but it means something very straightforward – ethical practice means that we are always looking for the best possible outcome for people in any given situation. Ethical standards mean that we want to protect, improve and empower the lives of children. This is not just about achieving a bare minimum, but about excelling. The questions below should also help you to reflect on ethical standards within your work. Again this will join with or impact on your personal standards and values.

- Can you name three features of the legislation on childcare for your country that may affect your work?

- If not, there are many books on the subject and it could be part of your group learning that you understand some elements of this in relation to children in care. Does anyone have a key text that they have really enjoyed reading or that provides access to information easily?

- What in your personal view is the most important aspect of safeguarding children in your daily work? What are the views of your team with regard to safeguarding children and what do you consider to be the most important area for safeguarding with regard to the particular child or young person in your care?

- What aspects of health and safety law do you feel are most significant to your work?

- What policies and procedures within your organisation do you consider most meaningful to your work on a daily basis? When did you last look at policies and procedures and when did you last ask anyone leading the organisation a question about their policies and procedures? If not – why not? What facility does your organisation have for questions to the leadership of your organisation?

- Can you name three Government policies which have directly affected your life or the lives of the children you care for (including your own children) in the last six months?

5. SIDE FIVE OF PENTAGON: EXPERT HELP AND THEORIES – DRAWING ON EXPERTISE AND CREATING NEW LEARNING OPPORTUNITIES

In this side of the Pentagon we are working towards the idea that we don't have all the answers in our own heads. We are working towards seeking out the knowledge of those who have gone before us, those who have made mistakes and learned from them, and those who work in other fields who may be able to help our understanding of being human. No single person will ever have all the answers. As a team we cannot have all of the answers but we can promote the idea of learning teams which means that you are learning something new all the time. This is more energising and exciting than a closed system where information is limited.

You may have one person in your team who is great on gathering theories and can hold these ideas for the rest of the team. You may have one person in the team who has a greater understanding of social pedagogy or therapeutic childcare and can explain this to the team as the idea unfolds. It does not have to be a complex theory. Another person in your team may have noticed that a child is more receptive when they are making cakes. That is a theory of your own, so go ahead and develop it for yourselves – make sponge cakes, scones, biscuits as often as you can, buy recipe books and spatulas and mixing bowls, cash in on the new learning opportunity for the child. If the activity has held their interest then you are going in the right direction. One child told me that he thought cognitive behavioural therapy was for dummies – the same child loved doing art work and craft with me and we made a beautiful necklace together for his Mum. We will often find that children will lead us to where they need to be if we listen intently.

However, there is no point in re-inventing the wheel. There are clear domains of knowledge that I would actively advise practitioners to learn about. There are some basic areas of knowledge such as understanding of communications skills, attachment theory, the effects of trauma, child development and motivational interviewing. However, don't be limited by this map. There is so much learning that can support you. An interest in politics and an understanding of democracy would assist you in your work. You may be interested in sport and outdoor pursuits and how this helps to develop children, or you may want to simply enjoy trying to create the best kind of environment for children both psychologically and emotionally as well as physically. Whatever your interest or domain of knowledge, it will be useful to your work.

6. THE CORE OF THE PENTAGON: WORKING TOGETHER – THE QUALITY OF RELATIONSHIP WE ARE ABLE TO FORM WITH THE CHILD

Finally we can turn the centre of our attention to the core of the Pentagon. We are looking here at the way we develop the relationship with the child or patient with whom we work. But it is also about the quality of the environment that we provide – the therapeutic milieu. We may not all be key players in the child's life and a child may relate to some people more easily than others. That does not mean that you may not play a key role in supporting the team to achieve the goals mentioned in Side one of the Pentagon (i.e. attention to the child). The therapeutic milieu could also be referred to as the atmosphere and environment that we provide.

This atmosphere has to be filled with possibility for change and opportunities to learn about behaviour. Every day has to be a new day in which a child can make a fresh start and learn successfully, even if the day before has been a disaster area. More important than learning will be the opportunity we provide for a child to feel safe and secure and feel nurtured and valued as an individual. The way that we prepare breakfast for the child, the way that we support them to tidy their room or encourage them to keep their clothes in good order, or talk them round from a bad mood, will all contribute to the changes that are needed. A colleague of mine referred to the environments that some children come from as a 'toxic soup'. This sounds dreadful but it is truly awful when a child comes from an environment where nobody cares about their well-being, nobody thinks about their social presentation, or the things they have to learn. Worse than that, they may come from an environment where acts may have been carried out that are intentionally harmful, neglectful and hurtful. What would you call that? This is referred to as being abusive and we have to be aware that we are transforming a child's consciousness gradually to the idea that environments can be beneficial, benign and enhancing and supportive rather than damaging. This can take a very long time to achieve and generally will take months and years rather than weeks. However, if you have the intention to help a child feel safe then you have the beginnings of a therapeutic milieu and a constructive relationship.

More than that if you can help a child reflect on their behaviour and gradually adapt to a positive environment and create positive emotional states, then you are creating the type of relationship that can be expected from therapeutic childcare – a relationship that helps a child to make changes. You could call that therapeutic if you wish, but you could just simply call it helpful. We are creating an environment in which children can integrate their states of mind and feel a sense of themselves as a whole, able to think, reflect and feel, and able to seek resolution to their fears and problems. The environment needs to tell this to the child as they live in it. A sign saying, 'We are here to help' could be useful, but your behaviour will signal to a child that you are willing to think with them and be supportive.

The Pentagon has been developed as a way to help carers and supporters to think ecologically about the environment that they provide for children. It is a visual aid that helps remind us of the task we have to achieve. Hopefully in reading through these pages you will have realised that the job of therapeutic childcare is more than a job – it is an opportunity to learn more about yourself so that you can support others more fully. The Pentagon is there as a prompt to help you question more deeply and observe more deeply all that you do in order to provide better outcomes for the children you care for.

Chapter 7

CONCLUSION

As human beings one of our strongest compulsions is the desire to create some certainty in our lives. This same tendency can also be one of the most inhibiting and detrimental forces to human development if things stay the same.

This is illustrated in Yann Martel's *Life of Pi* (2001) which has since been turned into an exquisitely beautiful film directed by Ang Lee. The narrator in the film lives in a zoo with his family in India and he is in effect a 'little philosopher' on life. He observes that there are people who do not approve of zoos because they think it is cruel to keep animals cooped up in cages and deprived of the freedom of nature. Actually he observes it is the very freedom and unpredictability of nature that animals and humans fear the most. Animals like to know when they are getting their next meal, and they spend a lot of time and invest a lot of energy in making sure that will happen.

As humans we are no different, being programmed to organise our world in the best possible way to ensure our survival. One way to avoid this overwhelming tendency to simply control and react to life from a fearful place, is to increase our capacity to reflect on and organise our experience so that we achieve the best state of continuance and the most refined solutions providing both continuity and stability, whilst at the same time giving room for growth, development and progress.

A tension also resides within the brain. We have the remarkable capacity to create and imagine with our so-called new or most recently developed brain. But we have tended to be defined by this new brain in our current age – it signals our identity as an individual and we are led by its tendency to achieve through active, goal-orientated behaviours. Yet this new brain and our individual identities are inextricably linked to an ancient and primitive brain with the desperate need to survive at all costs and to react to any threat combined with a desire to connect with others.

Whilst being subject to competing tendencies, we now know that our brains and consequently ourselves crave peace and harmony, and effective ways to relate. In this kind of social environment young people and children are trying to develop their identities and autonomy.

The competing demands made on both adults and children are complex. Whilst at first this may seem demanding and stressful, what it in fact requires is that we hone our psychological resources and use them to their best advantage.

We can achieve mindful solutions for children by using our brain to the best of its capability, and my proposal to you has been that we do this by sitting down quietly more often and for longer, taking time out for recovery and consideration of the facts that lay before us before we draw our conclusions and jump back into frenetic activity. Time out should become a legitimate act of the working day – used for reflective practice – rather than catching up on the 'to do' list.

It could be said that ticking boxes to monitor our behaviours at work is like owning a Rolls Royce, keeping it in the garage and cleaning it once a week to go to the shops. We have a brain that can do so much more than that – in our Rolls Royce brain we can travel in real style and go for long journeys; we can reach goals far more effectively if we use it. What is more, the whole organisation can get to ride in the Rolls Royce and the running costs are relatively cheap, requiring only good time management and commitment to the concept.

In this book I have tried to illustrate the meaning of reflective practice and mindfulness in therapeutic work with children so that you can see that it is a tool for effectiveness, sharpening interaction and giving meaning to difficulty. Once we give real meaning and understanding to the difficulty that a child is presenting to us, we are responding to the real needs of that child.

It is not a 'cure all' book about technique. Children need repeated patterns of soothing behaviour before they settle to the idea that life can be safe, but we will gain this outcome by starting on the journey to take time for reflective practice and allowing for the inexpensive luxury to think clearly about the meaning of the behaviours that we have to manage.

Ultimately you will find your own unique way to work with children who need your care and support. It is possible that by engaging in reflective practice as part of your work you can learn to transform the lives of children who are so very unhappy. Even in the most difficult and intransigent of cases, there is some hope of change. But we need to hold on to the idea that it is possible to create an environment in which we remain hopeful and thinking reflectively is certainly a way to do this. It is no miracle cure or quick fix, but we can at least create an environment in which we can think.

Sometimes all that can be contributed to a day is genuine authentic help with one more painful emotion or maybe the creation of one more helpful thought, but that is certainly worth the effort. Every time a child feels hope they will learn how to build hopeful lives in the future. Every time you are able to reflect on a difficult and painful experience with a child you care for so that you can make sense of it for them, you will have contributed to their development. You may only be showing a child some basic well-measured adult common sense to an everyday problem, but we must not underestimate the value of such an act on the development of a person. That may at times be the best we can do.

I hope that this book will guide you through the early stages of your reflective journey – until you can drive yourself.

APPENDIX
THE RIGHTS OF THE CHILD

Understanding the rights of the child is an important part of critical thinking and reflexivity (understanding how the world impacts on us). These are produced below to help develop an understanding of the impact of children's rights on our work. These were adopted by the United Nations General Assembly (resolution 1386) following the United Nations Convention on the Rights of the Child, where all children in the world were promised the same rights (although not all nations have adopted this Charter). However, these rights were developed by the United Nations as far back as December 1959.

Children who have been abused or harmed by adults have had their rights violated and therefore have a justified sense that the world is just not fair. They spend much time trying to right their sense that they are not equal to others – often not quite understanding the reasons why. In a previous article (North 2011) I have written that children who do not receive adequate and mindful parenting simply do not exist on an equal playing field to children who receive safe, thoughtful parenting. Therefore we cannot be surprised if they bear automatic grudges and even show themselves to be punitive towards others, at times for no reason. Inside they just feel that life has not been fair. The basis of the UN Charter is that children should be seen as developing individuals, they should be protected and shown respect and they should be given as a right the basic environment to support their development such as a decent home, food, clothing and education. The Charter respects the rights of parents to raise their own children in their own family environment according to their own codes and cultures. At the same time it places an emphasis on governments and authorities to take over and protect children if their rights are violated within the family environment.

The United Nations Convention on the Rights of the Child could be used as a therapeutic genre in its own right. When we train therapists and carers we ideally would have a module on the Rights of Children and consider each of the Articles involved. If you happen to work in a team who feel that they have a lull in their learning, you could go through the Charter and stimulate conversation and thinking about children and their rights. Equally if we help children to understand that they have rights but that they also have a responsibility to show respect for the rights of others, we can really help them by bringing fresh information to their thinking and perhaps promote discussion and change. Many boys I have worked with who are violent or even sexually abusive have no concept in their mind that they have violated the rights of others, because they have no concept of their own rights having been violated. They are just simply transferring their experiences onto others. They have had no help in reflection. If we can galvanise a child's innate sense of justice and fairness we can promote healing for them and at the same time turn them into responsible citizens.

You could also bear in mind that there are many children who are not going to want to talk about their life story or engage in therapeutic activities, because it is too frightening and threatening. However they may well engage with you in a reading of the facts about children's lives because these facts are indisputable. For this reason I have reproduced a child's version of the European Convention – written in simpler and less complicated language (see p.162). There are so many ways to work with this raw material. You could put up your own convention on the rights of children. Children could choose the Article that they like the most and make a poster to promote their new thinking. The Articles could be the centre of discussion and help children to think more clearly when and if they violate the rights of others. And the Charter just might give a child a sense that they want to talk with others about some of the thoughts and feelings that they have when they read it. This gives them a chance to project what is going on inside them into a discussion. It gives us further chances to show that we can be supportive and that we care about the way that children are treated.

The information reproduced below is taken from a fact sheet that is produced by UNICEF and further information is available at www.unicef.org/crc/files/Rights_overview.pdf.

Article 1 (Definition of the child): The Convention defines a 'child' as a person below the age of 18, unless the laws of a particular country set the legal age for adulthood younger. The Committee on the Rights of the Child, the monitoring body for the Convention, has encouraged States to review the age of majority if it is set below 18 and to increase the level of protection for all children under 18.

Article 2 (Non-discrimination): The Convention applies to all children, whatever their race, religion or abilities; whatever they think or say, whatever type of family they come from. It doesn't matter where children live, what language they speak, what their parents do, whether they are boys or girls, what their culture is, whether they have a disability or whether they are rich or poor. No child should be treated unfairly on any basis.

Article 3 (Best interests of the child): The best interests of children must be the primary concern in making decisions that may affect them. All adults should do what is best for children. When adults make decisions, they should think about how their decisions will affect children. This particularly applies to budget, policy and law makers.

Article 4 (Protection of rights): Governments have a responsibility to take all available measures to make sure children's rights are respected, protected and fulfilled. When countries ratify the Convention, they agree to review their laws relating to children. This involves assessing their social services, legal, health and educational systems, as well as levels of funding for these services. Governments are then obliged to take all necessary steps to ensure that the minimum standards set by the Convention in these areas are being met. They must help families protect children's rights and create an environment where they can grow and reach their potential. In some instances, this may involve changing existing laws or creating new ones. Such legislative changes are not imposed, but come about through the same process by which any law is created or reformed within a country. Article 41 of the Convention points out that when a country already has higher legal standards than those seen in the Convention, the higher standards always prevail.

Article 5 (Parental guidance): Governments should respect the rights and responsibilities of families to direct and guide their children so that, as they grow, they learn to use their rights properly. Helping children to understand their rights does not mean pushing them to make choices with consequences that they are too young to handle. Article 5 encourages parents to deal with rights issues 'in a manner consistent with the evolving capacities of the child'. The Convention does not take responsibility for children away from their parents and give more authority to governments. It does place on governments the responsibility to protect and assist families in fulfilling their essential role as nurturers of children.

Article 6 (Survival and development): Children have the right to live. Governments should ensure that children survive and develop healthily.

Article 7 (Registration, name, nationality, care): All children have the right to a legally registered name, officially recognised by the government. Children have the right to a nationality (to belong to a country). Children also have the right to know and, as far as possible, to be cared for by their parents.

Article 8 (Preservation of identity): Children have the right to an identity – an official record of who they are. Governments should respect children's right to a name, a nationality and family ties.

Article 9 (Separation from parents): Children have the right to live with their parent(s), unless it is bad for them. Children whose parents do not live together have the right to stay in contact with both parents, unless this might hurt the child.

Article 10 (Family reunification): Families whose members live in different countries should be allowed to move between those countries so that parents and children can stay in contact, or get back together as a family.

Article 11 (Kidnapping): Governments should take steps to stop children being taken out of their own country illegally. This article is particularly concerned with parental abductions. The Convention's Optional Protocol on the sale of children, child prostitution and child pornography has a provision that concerns abduction for financial gain.

Article 12 (Respect for the views of the child): When adults are making decisions that affect children, children have the right to say what they think should happen and have their opinions taken into account.

This does not mean that children can now tell their parents what to do. This Convention encourages adults to listen to the opinions of children and involve them in decision-making – not give children authority over adults. Article 12 does not interfere with parents' right and responsibility to express their views on matters affecting their children. Moreover, the Convention recognises that the level of a child's participation in decisions must be appropriate to the child's level of maturity. Children's ability to form and express their opinions develops with age and most adults will naturally give the views of teenagers greater weight than those of a pre-schooler, whether in family, legal or administrative decisions.

Article 13 (Freedom of expression): Children have the right to get and share information, as long as the information is not damaging to them or others. In exercising the right to freedom of expression, children have the responsibility to also respect the rights, freedoms and reputations of others. The freedom of expression includes the right to share information in any way they choose, including by talking, drawing or writing.

Article 14 (Freedom of thought, conscience and religion): Children have the right to think and believe what they want and to practise their religion, as long as they are not stopping other people from enjoying their rights. Parents should help guide their children in these matters. The Convention respects the rights and duties of parents in providing religious and moral guidance to their children. Religious groups around the world have expressed support for the Convention, which indicates that it in no way prevents parents from bringing their children up within a religious tradition. At the same time, the Convention recognises that as children mature and are able to form their own views, some may question certain religious practices or cultural traditions. The Convention supports children's right to examine their beliefs, but it also states that their right to express their beliefs implies respect for the rights and freedoms of others.

Article 15 (Freedom of association): Children have the right to meet together and to join groups and organisations, as long as it does not stop other people from enjoying their rights. In exercising their rights, children have the responsibility to respect the rights, freedoms and reputations of others.

Article 16 (Right to privacy): Children have a right to privacy. The law should protect them from attacks against their way of life, their good name, their families and their homes.

Article 17 (Access to information; mass media):
Children have the right to get information that is important to their health and well-being. Governments should encourage mass media – radio, television, newspapers and Internet content sources – to provide information that children can understand and to not promote materials that could harm children. Mass media should particularly be encouraged to supply information in languages that minority and indigenous children can understand. Children should also have access to children's books.

Article 18 (Parental responsibilities; state assistance):
Both parents share responsibility for bringing up their children, and should always consider what is best for each child. Governments must respect the responsibility of parents for providing appropriate guidance to their children – the Convention does not take responsibility for children away from their parents and give more authority to governments. It places a responsibility on governments to provide support services to parents, especially if both parents work outside the home.

Article 19 (Protection from all forms of violence):
Children have the right to be protected from being hurt and mistreated, physically or mentally. Governments should ensure that children are properly cared for and protect them from violence, abuse and neglect by their parents, or anyone else who looks after them. In terms of discipline, the Convention does not specify what forms of punishment parents should use. However, any form of discipline involving violence is unacceptable. There are ways to discipline children that are effective in helping children learn about family and social expectations for their behaviour – those that are non-violent, are appropriate to

the child's level of development and take the best interests of the child into consideration. In most countries, laws already define what sorts of punishments are considered excessive or abusive. It is up to each government to review these laws in light of the Convention.

Article 20 (Children deprived of family environment): Children who cannot be looked after by their own family have a right to special care and must be looked after properly, by people who respect their ethnic group, religion, culture and language.

Article 21 (Adoption): Children have the right to care and protection if they are adopted or in foster care. The first concern must be what is best for them. The same rules should apply whether they are adopted in the country where they were born, or if they are taken to live in another country.

Article 22 (Refugee children): Children have the right to special protection and help if they are refugees (if they have been forced to leave their home and live in another country), as well as all the rights in this Convention.

Article 23 (Children with disabilities): Children who have any kind of disability have the right to special care and support, as well as all the rights in the Convention, so that they can live full and independent lives.

Article 24 (Health and health services): Children have the right to good quality health care – the best health care possible – to safe drinking water, nutritious food, a clean and safe environment, and information to help them stay healthy. Rich countries should help poorer countries achieve this.

Article 25 (Review of treatment in care): Children who are looked after by their local authorities, rather than their parents, have the right to have these living arrangements looked at regularly to see if they are the most appropriate. Their care and treatment should always be based on 'the best interests of the child'. (See Guiding Principles, Article 3.)

Article 26 (Social security): Children – either through their guardians or directly – have the right to help from the government if they are poor or in need.

Article 27 (Adequate standard of living): Children have the right to a standard of living that is good enough to meet their physical and mental needs. Governments should help families and guardians who cannot afford to provide this, particularly with regard to food, clothing and housing.

Article 28: (Right to education): All children have the right to a primary education, which should be free. Wealthy countries should help poorer countries achieve this right. Discipline in schools should respect children's dignity. For children to benefit from education, schools must be run in an orderly way – without the use of violence. Any form of school discipline should take into account the child's human dignity. Therefore, governments must ensure that school administrators review their discipline policies and eliminate any discipline practices involving physical or mental violence, abuse or neglect. The Convention places a high value on education. Young people should be encouraged to reach the highest level of education of which they are capable.

Article 29 (Goals of education): Children's education should develop each child's personality, talents and abilities to the fullest. It should encourage children to respect others, human rights and their own and other cultures. It should also help them learn to live peacefully, protect the environment and respect other people. Children have a particular responsibility to respect the rights of their parents, and education should aim to develop respect for the values and culture of their parents.

Article 30 (Children of minorities/indigenous groups): Minority or indigenous children have the right to learn about and practice their own culture, language and religion. The right to practice one's own culture, language and religion applies to everyone; the Convention here highlights this right in instances where the practices are not shared by the majority of people in the country.

Article 31 (Leisure, play and culture): Children have the right to relax and play, and to join in a wide range of cultural, artistic and other recreational activities.

Article 32 (Child labour): The government should protect children from work that is dangerous or might harm their health or their education. While the Convention protects children from harmful and exploitative work, there is nothing in it that prohibits parents from expecting their children to help out at home in ways that are safe and appropriate to their age. If children help out in a family farm or business, the tasks they do should be safe and suited to their level of development and comply with national labour laws. Children's work should not jeopardise any of their other rights, including the right to education, or the right to relaxation and play.

Article 33 (Drug abuse): Governments should use all means possible to protect children from the use of harmful drugs and from being used in the drug trade.

Article 34 (Sexual exploitation): Governments should protect children from all forms of sexual exploitation and abuse.

Article 35 (Abduction, sale and trafficking): The government should take all measures possible to make sure that children are not abducted, sold or trafficked.

Article 36 (Other forms of exploitation): Children should be protected from any activity that takes advantage of them or could harm their welfare and development.

Article 37 (Detention and punishment): No one is allowed to punish children in a cruel or harmful way. Children who break the law should not be treated cruelly. They should not be put in prison with adults, should be able to keep in contact with their families, and should not be sentenced to death or life imprisonment without possibility of release.

Article 38 (War and armed conflicts): Governments must do everything they can to protect and care for children affected by war. Children under 15 should not be forced or recruited to take part in a war or join the armed forces. The Convention's Optional Protocol on the involvement of children in armed conflict further develops this right, raising the age for direct participation in armed conflict to 18 and establishing a ban on compulsory recruitment for children under 18.

Article 39 (Rehabilitation of child victims): Children who have been neglected, abused or exploited should receive special help to physically and psychologically recover and reintegrate into society. Particular attention should be paid to restoring the health, self-respect and dignity of the child.

Article 40 (Juvenile justice): Children who are accused of breaking the law have the right to legal help and fair treatment in a justice system that respects their rights. Governments are required to set a minimum age below which children cannot be held criminally responsible and to provide minimum guarantees for the fairness and quick resolution of judicial or alternative proceedings.

Article 41 (Respect for superior national standards): If the laws of a country provide better protection of children's rights than the articles in this Convention, those laws should apply.

Article 42 (Knowledge of rights): Governments should make the Convention known to adults and children. Adults should help children learn about their rights, too. (See also Article 4.)

Articles 43–54 (implementation measures): These articles discuss how governments and international organisations like UNICEF should work to ensure children are protected in their rights.

RIGHTS FOR CHILDREN – WRITTEN FROM A CHILD'S PERSPECTIVE

As a child you have rights. These are things you can expect from people:

1. If you are under 18 you are still a child or if you are a teenager you are a young person. There are things you can expect from the way that people behave towards you. You should be treated fairly at all times and you should feel that you can then treat others fairly.

2. It does not matter where you live or what language you speak or what colour your skin is. It does not matter if you are a boy or a girl or what your culture is or whether you are rich or poor or what has happened to you in your life or which religion you were born to. You should be treated fairly and kindly by people. This is also called respect. We should expect to receive this as well as to give it to others.

3. Adults who care for you should do what is best for you – they should also tell you what they are doing to help you so that you know what is happening. You should feel you can ask questions about things happening in your life at any time.

4. You should be able to ask your parent or social worker or person who cares for you about the laws that are made to help children and how people should be treating you.

5. The people who care for you (whether they are your parents or not) should support you to make good decisions for yourself too. This is because you

are young and have to rely on them for support and information about the world – adults are there to help you – not to harm you.

6. All adults should be helping you to live a good life; this includes people in your community as well as people who look after you and parents. If people are not helping you or they are harming you – you should find someone to tell. People should always help you to do the right thing or act in the right way.

7. You have the right to see important pieces of paper that are all about you, such as your birth certificate and passport. You need to know which country you belong to. You have the right to know your real name and about your birth family.

8. You have the right to be cared for by your parents unless they cannot do this properly, in which case you have the right to be cared for by a caring person but you have the right to know who your parents are. If your parents are separated you have the right to stay in contact with both parents unless this might hurt you. If your parents live in different countries you should be able to stay in contact.

9. You should not be taken out of your own country illegally. If this happens it is called abduction or kidnapping. If anyone does this to you – you should tell someone you can trust straight away or as soon as it is safe.

10. You have the right to have your say in decisions that matter to you and your ideas should be taken into consideration. That does not mean that you can tell

your parents or people who care for you what to do all the time, but it does mean that they should listen to what you think.

11. You should be able to share your honest thoughts and feelings with people. This includes talking, drawing or writing.

12. You have the right to think and believe what you want. You can practice your religion and you must help others to enjoy their rights to their own religion. We have to respect others too.

13. You have the right to meet with other children and join groups and organisations.

14. You have a right to privacy and to be alone when you want that.

15. You have the right to get information that is important to your life and health. Adults should help you with this and if you cannot read you have the right to ask for help with this. If you cannot understand you should feel free to tell people so that they can help you.

16. You have the right to be protected from being hurt and mistreated physically or mentally. If people discipline you to help you to understand something you have done wrong, it must be fair and must not be harmful in any way but simply be part of helping you to understand. Discipline should not be harmful.

17. Children who cannot be looked after by their own family have a right to special care and must be looked after properly by people who respect their ethnic group, religion, culture and language.

18. Children have the right to care and protection if they are adopted or in foster care. The first concern must be what is best for them. If the Local Authority cares for you the foster parents or carers should be inspected regularly to see if the care is good.

19. Children have the right to special protection and help if they are refugees from another country.

20. Children with disability have the right to special care and support so that they can live full and independent lives.

21. Children have the right to health care, good drinking water, nutritious food and a clean safe environment. Your standard of living should meet your needs.

22. Children have the right to support from their Local Authority if they are poor or in need.

23. All children have the right to a primary education which should be free. School discipline should take into account your dignity. You should develop your best talents to the fullest.

24. Children in minority groups have the right to practise and learn about their own culture, language or religion. You should not be afraid just because there are not many people like you. You should be proud to be different.

25. Children have the right to relax and play and to join in a wide range of activities like art, music, dance, theatre or sport.

26. The government should protect children from work that is dangerous or might harm their health. Children should not be exploited for labour.

27. Adults and governments should do everything possible to protect children from drug abuse, sexual exploitation and abduction. They should protect and care for children affected by war.

28. No one is allowed to punish a child in a cruel or harmful way. People should help you to do the right thing if you have got something wrong. They should do this by talking to you but not physically punishing you.

29. Children who have been neglected, abused or exploited or treated badly should receive special help to recover and reintegrate into society. Attention should be paid to helping you get back your health and self-respect and most of all your happiness and enjoyment of life.

30. Adults should help children to learn about their rights.

BIBLIOGRAPHY

Alvesson, M. and Skoldberg, K. (2000) *Reflexive Methodology: New Vistas for Qualitative Research.* London: Sage Publications.

Baron Cohen, S. (2001) 'Autistic spectrum disorder.' *Journal of Autism and Developmental Disorders 31*, 5, 31–35.

Bowlby, J. (1951) 'Maternal Care and Mental Health'. *Bulletin of the World Health Organisation 3*, 335–534.

Bowlby, J. (1953) *Childcare and the Growth of Love.* London: Penguin.

Bowlby, J. (1988) *A Secure Base.* London: Routledge Classics.

Bowlby, J. (1990) *Charles Darwin: A New Life.* London: Norton Publishing.

Brach, T. (2003) *Radical Acceptance: Embracing your Life with the Heart of a Buddha.* New York: Bantam Publishing.

Cohen, N.J., Muire, E., Lojkasek, M., Muire, R., Parker, C.J., Barwick, M. and Brown, M. (1999) 'Watch, wait and wonder: testing the effectiveness of a new approach to mother infant psychotherapy.' *Infant Mental Health Journal 20*, 4, 429–451.

Darwin, C. (1859) *The Origin of Species and The Voyage of The Beagle.* Everyman's New York: Library.

Department for Education (2003) *Every Child Matters.* United Kingdom Green Paper. London: HMSO. Available at www.education.gov. uk/consultations/downloadableDocs/EveryChildMatters.pdf, accessed 2 September 2013.

DSM IV (2000) *Diagnostic and Statistical Manual of Mental Disorders*, 4th edn. Washington, DC: American Psychiatric Association.

Flavell, J.H. (1999) 'Cognitive development: children's knowledge about the mind.' *Annual Review of Psychology 50*, 9, 21–45.

Fonagy, P. (2004) *Psychotherapy for Borderline Personality Disorder: Mentalization Based Treatment with Anthony Bateman.* Oxford: Oxford University Press.

Fonagy P. and Target, M. (1997) 'Attachment and reflective function: their role in self organisation.' *Development and Psychopathology 9*, 4, 679–700.

Fonagy, P., Gergely, G., Jurist, E.L. and Target, M. (2004) *Affect Regulation, Mentalization, and the Development of the Self.* London and New York: Karnac.

Fosha, D., Siegel, D.J. and Solomon, M. (2009) *The Healing Power of Emotion: Affective Neuroscience, Development and Clinical Practice.* London: W.W. Norton.

Gilbert, P. (2010) *The Compassionate Mind.* London: Constable.

Griffin, J. and Tyrrell, I. (2011) *Human Givens: A New Approach to Emotional Health and Clear Thinking.* Chalvington: HG Publishing.

Hawkins, P. and Shohet, R. (1989) *Supervision in the Helping Professions.* Milton Keynes: Open University Press.

Hodges, J., Steele., M., Hillman, S., Henderson, K. and Kaniuk, J. (2003) 'Changes in attachment representations over the first year of adoptive placement: narratives of maltreated children.' *Clinical Child Psychology and Psychiatry 8*, 3, 351–367.

Holloway, E. (1995) *Clinical Supervision: A Systems Approach.* Los Angeles, CA: Sage Publications.

Hughes, D.A. (1998) *Facilitating Developmental Attachment: The Road to Emotional Recovery and Behavioral Change in Foster and Adopted Children.* Lanham, MD: Aronson.

ICD-10 (1993) *Classification of Mental and Behavioural Disorders: Diagnostic Criteria for Research.* Geneva: World Health Organization.

Kabat Zinn, J. (2012) *Mindfulness for Beginners.* Louisville, CO: Sounds True Books.

Kipling, R. (1895) *'If' Poem in Complete Works of Rudyard Kipling.* London: Delphi Classics.

Leitch, R. (2008) 'Lecture by Dr Ruth Leitch of Quenn's University Belfast, May, 2008, "Creative Methodologies" at Metanoia Institute London.' Ealing, London: Metanoia Institute.

Martel, Y. (2001) *Life of Pi.* New York: Knopf.

Maslow, A.H. (1943) 'A theory of human motivation.' *Psychological Review 50*, 4, 370–396.

North, J. (2010) *How to Think About Caring for a Child with Difficult Behaviour*. Exmouth: Watershed.

North, J. 'Working with the State as Parent.' *BACP Children and Young People*, May, 2011, 14–16.

Rogers, C.R. (1961) *On Becoming a Person*. London: Constable Publishing.

Rollnick, S. and Miller, W. (1991) *Motivational Interviewing: Helping People Change*. New York and London: Guilford Press.

Revans, R. (2011) *The ABC of Action Learning*. Aldershot: Gower Publishing.

Schore, A.N. (1994) *Affect Regulation and the Origin of the Self: The Neurobiology of Emotional Development, Protocols and Procedures*. New York: Guilford Press.

Schon, D.A. (1991) *The Reflective Practitioner: How Professionals Think in Action*. Farnham: Ashgate Press.

Senge, P., Kleiner, A., Roberts, C., Ross, R., Roth, G. and Smith, B. (1999) *The Dance of Change: The Challenges of Sustaining Momentum in Learning Organizations*. New York: Doubleday/Currency.

Siegel D.J. (2007) *The Mindful Brain*. London: Norton.

Siegel D.J. (2010a) *The Mindful Therapist: A Clinician's Guide to Mindsight and Neural Integration*. London: Norton.

Siegel, D.J. (2010b) *Mindsight: The Science of Personal Transformation*. London: Random House Publishing.

Siegel, D.J. (2011) *The Whole Brain Child*. London: Random House Publishing.

Siegel D.J. (2012a) *The Pocket Guide to Interpersonal Neurobiology: An Integrative Handbook of The Mind*. London: Norton.

Siegel, D.J. (2012b) *The Developing Mind*, 2nd edn. London: Norton.

Sroufe, L.A., Egeland, B., Carlson, E.A. and Collins, W.A. (2005a) *The Development of the Person*. New York: Guilford.

Sroufe, L.A., DeHart, G.B. and Cooper, R.G. (2005b) *Child Development: Its Nature and Course*, 5th edn. London: McGraw Hill.

Stern, D.N. (1998) *The Interpersonal World of the Infant: A View from Psychoanalysis and Developmental Psychology*. London: Karnac.

United Nations Convention on the Rights of the Child (1989) Available at www.unicef.org/crc/index_30160.html, accessed on 03 July 2013.

Watzlawick, P. (1978) *The Language of Change.* London: Norton.

Williams, M., Teasdale, J., Segal, Z. and Kabat-Zinn, J. (2007) *The Mindful Way Through Depression: Freeing Yourself from Chronic Unhappiness.* New York: Guilford Press.

INDEX

abandonment 34, 105
abuse 69, 76, 90–1, 133,
    142
  in local authority care
    105
acceptance 34, 35
achievements 110, 114–16
Action Learning 15
actualisation 110
adaptation 15, 41, 53, 87,
    142
*Affect Regulation and the Origin
    of the Self* 40
aggression
  and excessive control 111
  and lack of protection
    112
  and poor communication
    skills 32
  as source of stress in
    teams 128
  assisting children to learn
    from 119
  in TV/computer games
    66, 67
  passive 76
  resolved through shift in
    thinking 58–9
  see also anger
anger 25, 75, 102
  management 116, 126
  see also aggression
anxiety
  about economic survival
    86
  acceptance of own 34
  and conflict 127
  and difficult behaviour
    81
  and information sharing
    75
  and predictability 71

and the limbic system 66
assessment of child's 101
awareness of own 43, 52
inability to express 56
in attachment 9
in relating to others 95
resolution through
    pretend play 63
resulting from
    disharmony 40
argument 81, 82
art 17, 22, 23, 29
assumptions 31, 78, 100,
    102–3, 106
attachment 9, 92, 94,
    106–9
  see also attachment theory
attachment model of
    personal development
    15
attachment theory 17, 82,
    85, 113, 140
  see also attachment
attention 40, 46, 63, 84,
    94, 110
  reparative 47
attitudes 7, 12, 94, 116
attunement 62–3
authenticity 26, 79
authority 12, 31, 86, 111,
    128
Autism Research Centre 28
autistic spectrum disorders
    27–8
autobiographical memory
    85
autonomy 31, 110, 146
awareness 13, 45, 50, 79,
    82, 117, 123, 134

balance 40
Baron-Cohen, Simon 28

behaviour
  and experiences 92
  and inner life 102
  challenging/difficult
    21, 55, 81, 84–5,
    111–12
  closed 132
  complex 10
  dysfunctional 24
  incoherent 47
  management of 13, 116
  modelling of expectations
    through 12
  reflection on 142
  understanding 100
  unconscious 53
'being brain' 61
beliefs 12, 82, 95, 119–20
blaming 132–3
blind spots 131
blitz, the 88
blocked thinking 55–60
body, the 44–8
  awareness of 50
bowel problems 56
Bowlby, John 14, 15, 17,
    80, 82, 85
brain development 21–2
breathing 44, 54
Buddhism 37
bullying 129, 133

capabilities 106
carers
  aggressive interactions
    with 58
  and complex behaviours
    10
  and developmental
    changes in children
    72